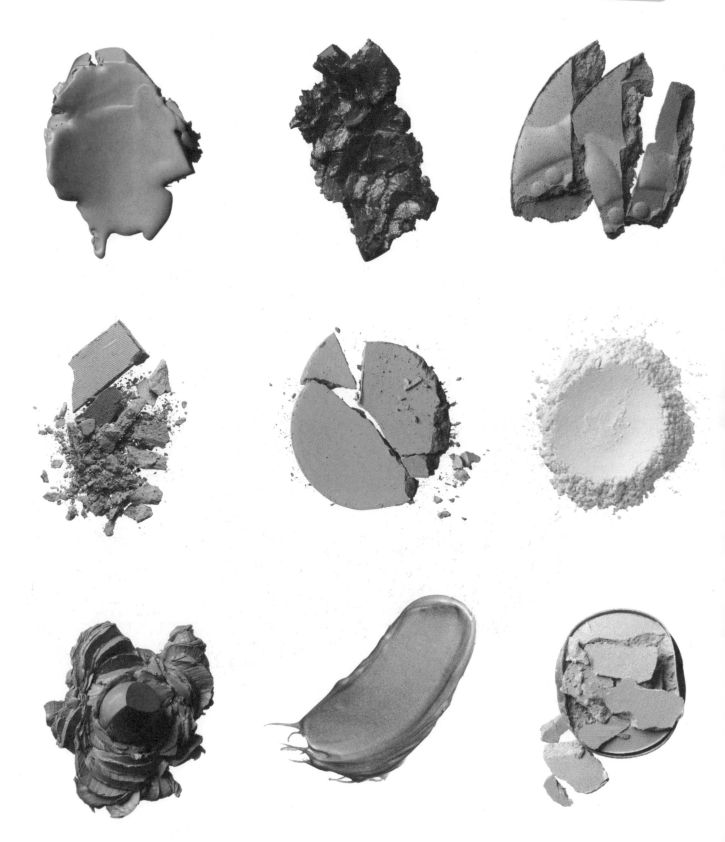

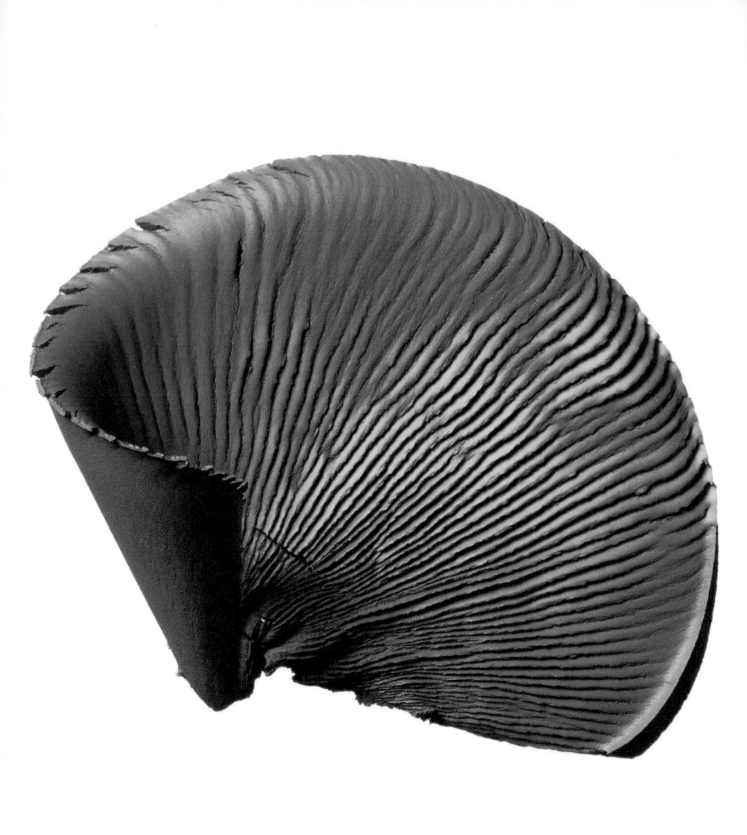

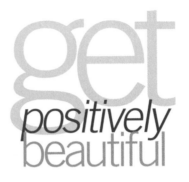

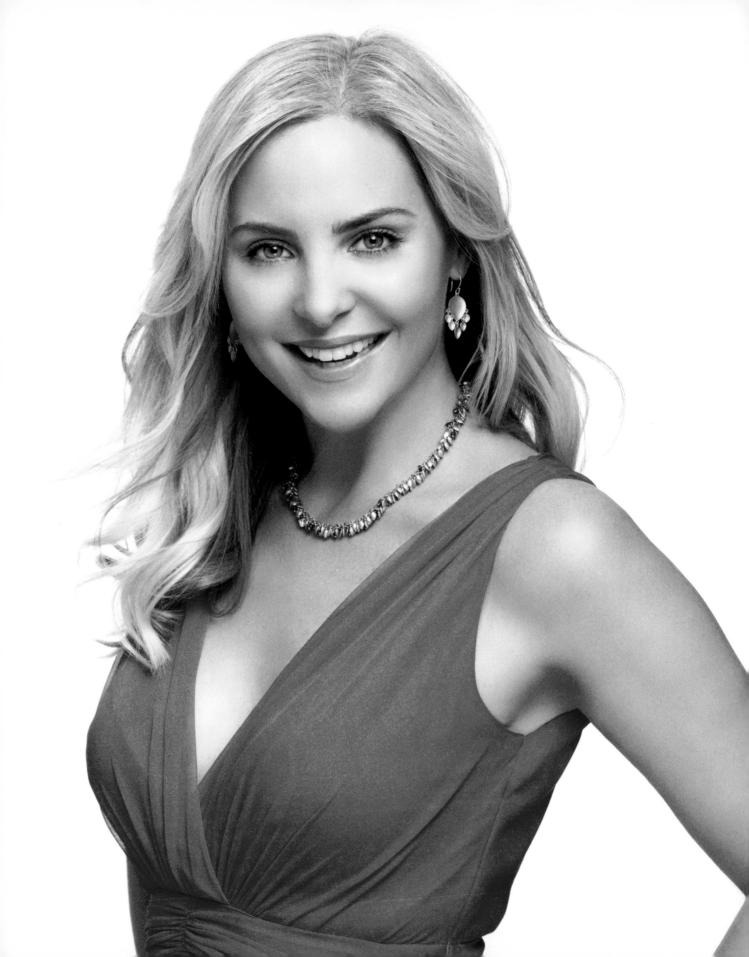

get *positively* beautiful

the ultimate guide to looking and feeling gorgeous

carmindy

CENTER
STREET®

New York Boston Nashville

Also by Carmindy
The 5-Minute Face:
The Quick & Easy Makeup Guide for Every Woman

Cover and Beauty Photography by Peter Buckingham
Still-Life Photography by Devon Jarvis
Hair by Noah Hatton
Styling by Lulu Chen
Dress by Miguelina
Jewelry by Me&Ro
Illustrations by Aimee Levy for Art Department

Center Street
Hachette Book Group USA
237 Park Avenue
New York, NY 10017
Visit our Web site at www.centerstreet.com.

Center Street is a division of Hachette Book Group USA, Inc. The Center Street name and logo are trademarks of Hachette Book Group USA, Inc.

Printed in the United States of America

First Edition: October 2008

10 9 8 7 6 5 4 3 2 1

Library of Congress Cataloging-in-Publication Data
Carmindy.
Get positively beautiful: the ultimate guide to looking and feeling gorgeous / Carmindy. — 1st ed.
   p. cm.
ISBN-13: 978-1-59995-143-0
ISBN-10: 1-59995-143-6
1. Beauty, Personal. 2. Face—Care and hygiene. 3. Skin—Care and hygiene. 4. Cosmetics. I. Title.
RA778.C21674 2008
646.7'2--dc22   2008017814

Design by Roger Gorman, Reiner Design NYC

To my loving husband, Javier, who has always made me feel like the most beautiful woman in the world.

Te amo, mi vida.

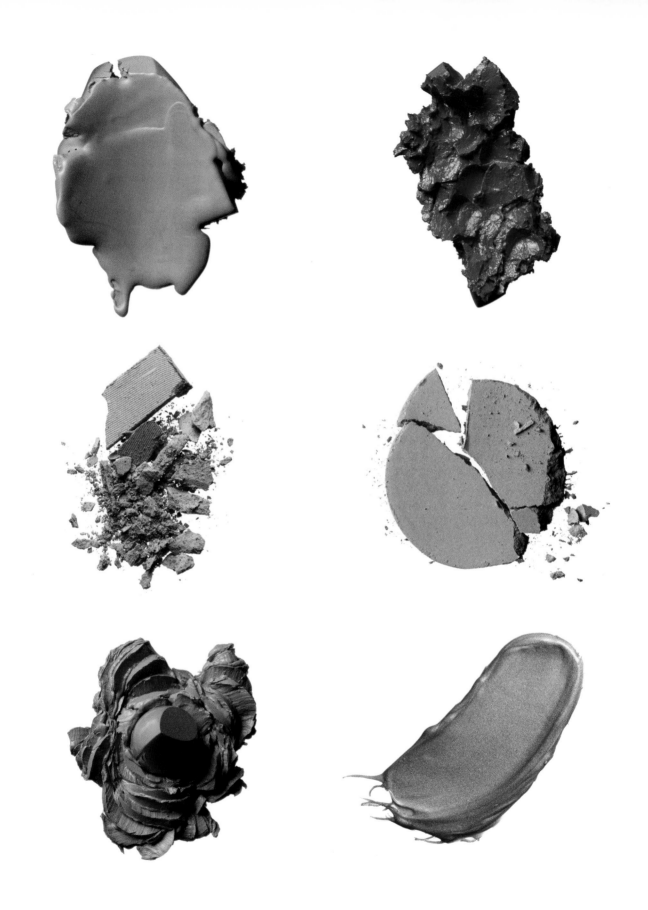

contents

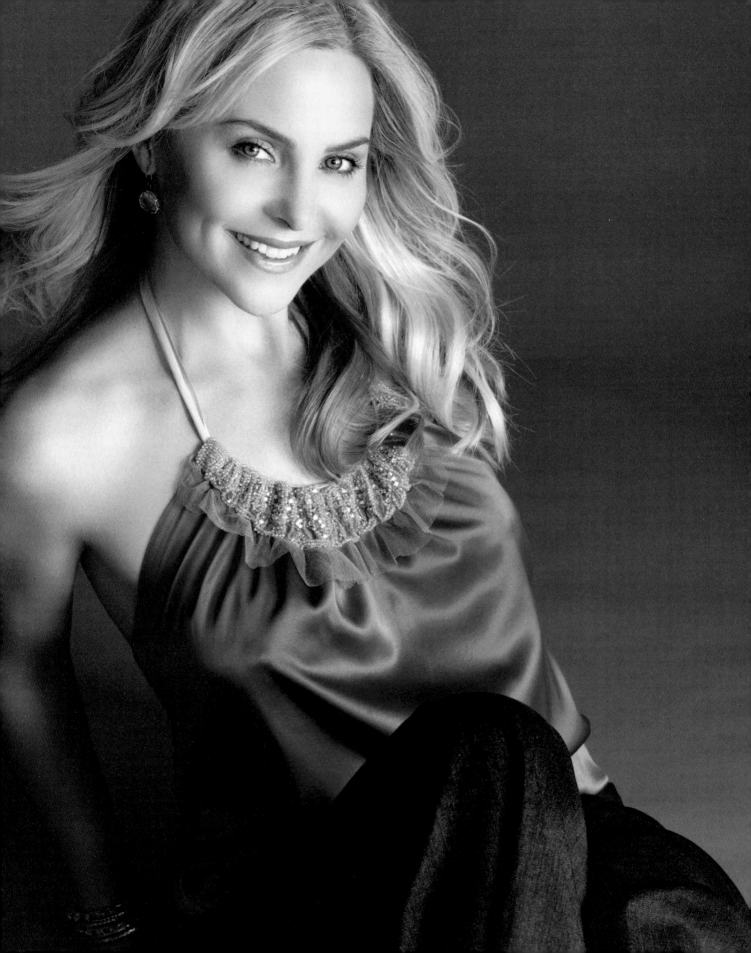

If everyone were cast in the same mold, there would be no such thing as beauty.
—CHARLES DARWIN

chapter one first things **first**

I believe looking good starts with feeling good.

Before we consider what to put on our faces, we must confront what's going on inside our heads! For a lot of us, it's a blurry mess of negativity. But right now, we can choose to make a change: we can decide to sharpen our focus and start seeing the positive.

I hear the skeptics out there already. *Hey, Carmindy, that's great and everything, but could you just show me how to make my lips look bigger?* Well, guess what? I can show you lots of ways to gloss up your pucker, but you'll only be pretty if you feel that way without a darn thing on those lips. And you'll only *be* beautiful when kind, loving words pass from them!

Words are incredibly powerful, and thoughts are even more so. Need proof?

How often have you stopped a friend whose eyes were clouded with worry and said, "What's the matter? You look upset." Or conversely, you've seen that same friend floating on cloud nine and said, "You look amazing. What's going on?" Same woman, different thoughts—a totally altered appearance.

That dynamic plays out on our own faces every day. How we think affects how we look. Period.

Though we can't always control how the world comes at us, we *can* decide to feel good about ourselves and to meet challenges head-on, with our best face forward. A confident face that knows its finest features and plays them up. A one-of-a-kind face that honors its special beauty and *owns* it from the inside out.

I've built my career by homing in on the natural beauty I find in each woman I consult with. But do you know what I spend the most time doing? It isn't mascara. It's convincing a woman to see the gorgeous potential I see in her and to *believe* in her own gifts.

Fans of *What Not to Wear* know how stubborn I can be about this. I simply won't allow a capable, captivating woman to sit before me and tear herself down. How can I consider a makeover a success if a lady hasn't first made over her mind? This goes especially for you, my friend!

You chose this book because you want to bring out your best. It's such a privilege for me to play a part in your transformation. And so exciting! Let's get going by turning off those negative old thought patterns and switching on the lovely light you *know* is burning inside.

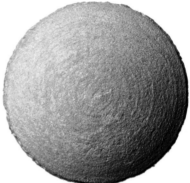

Here's how . . .

Drop the Flaw Focus

Sounds simple, right? But after two decades in the beauty biz, I know how difficult it is to shut out the negative messages coming at us every day.

Think for a moment about beauty "experts" who show us how to fix what they perceive is wrong with a given face. They see and point out the flaws first—expecting us to agree with the criticism—and then give instruction on how to camouflage the "issue." We can get so caught up in obeying their authority that we start transferring other women's "problem areas" to our own faces: suddenly we can only see dark undereye circles or thin lips. Before you know it, we feel worse than before.

We can hardly place blame on the beauty industry alone. Often the destructive cycle starts much closer to home.

No matter who you are, chances are people in your past have made negative comments about your appearance. Maybe a childhood bully yelled, "Hey, pizza face." Or an uncle whispered, "Quite a honker of a schnoz she's got there." Or a controlling boyfriend hissed, "Your eyes are so tiny, no wonder you can't drive straight."

I'm sure you have your own painful list. Why is it that we remember the insults and forget the compliments? Beats me, but we do—especially when we're young and forming our ideas about ourselves, and looking to others for guidance. When people close to us try to boost their self-importance by cutting us down, the wounds go deep.

Again, it's all about the power of words. We hold on to these negative opinions as truth. A nasty remark said in passing turns into a long-lasting insecurity. Rather than fight the insults, we agree. What's worse is that we take over the role of critic and turn up the volume.

I can't tell you how many women I have worked with who, when I say, "Wow, what beautiful eyes you have," argue that they are too small. Or if I say, "Check out your terrific complexion," they'll point out how big their pores are. I feel like calling the Centers for Disease Control to report an epidemic of facial dysmorphic disorder!

Even if you have been lucky enough to go through life unscathed by negative comments, you may have chosen to generate your own, perhaps as a member of the age-hating party. You may be one of those women who tracks every miniscule change, scrutinizing and agonizing. Every trip to the mirror ends in panicked dread.

It's ridiculous. It's also a serious misuse of our feminine power.

By focusing on what's "wrong" with our looks, we're—by definition—dwelling on the negative. When we're harsh with ourselves, we're agreeing with those who sought to hurt us. And we're fueling a damaging cycle that not only dulls our appearance but also darkens our days. Now I ask you, is that how we want to be? Acting as our own worst enemies?

I hear you, feisty ladies. *N.O.*

So, what do we say *yes* to instead? Being positively beautiful by celebrating our individuality and enhancing our unique assets.

Every woman has a special bloom all her own. Now is the time to take notice—starting in our own mirrors.

I realize your urge might be to fight me on this. Old habits are tough to break. But has being so tough on yourself brought you the results you want? Clearly not.

By dropping the flaw focus, you set off on a new path, one that's freeing and wonderful.

To understand how silly it is to hold one standard of beauty and to see any variation from it as a flaw, play along with me for a moment . . .

Imagine hearing a floral expert on a home improvement show proclaiming, "*Only* roses are beautiful." Our instincts would disagree. But, hey, we might still listen. A few minutes later, some of us might believe it and consider tearing up our magnolia trees and painting our orchids to look like roses. But why stop there? Delicate violets, striking birds of paradise? Hit the trash. Elegant calla lilies, scentsational lilacs? Off you go. Heck, we might grow to resent the rose's beauty and stop caring about flowers altogether. How absurd, right? Well, we have spent far too much time plucking away at *our* petals, and it has to stop.

Let go of the past. Drop that destructive commentary stuck on repeat. It's a tired track, and no one can dance to it!

How?

Start by trying this simple exercise. Look into a mirror and speak aloud your usual negative thoughts, like, "Ugh. These dark circles." Notice your whole facial expression as you say it. Now take a deep breath, concentrate on something positive in the same area, and praise it, loud and proud. "Check out my gorgeous eyes." What happens to your face simply from switching your focus and your words?

I'd bet my bottom dollar you immediately look happier, more relaxed. Now, does it feel a little silly at first? Maybe. But it's a whole lot sillier to be dishing yourself a big ol' plate of negative energy that manifests itself right smack in the middle of your face. Speaking sweetly of yourself, to yourself is more than a nicety. It's a necessity and the most potent beauty secret I know.

Ultimately, it's up to you to let go and take that first step toward the positive. You're in charge of your thoughts and emotions. It's your face, your image, and your life. Do you want it to be about your flaws or about your fabulousness?

Exactly.

Kick Away Corrosive Comparisons

Getting your mind made up to be beauty-positive is a fantastic first step. But staying focused on your unique attributes requires constant care, especially when the media and advertisers conspire to sabotage our efforts by inviting us to play the most time-wasting game ever: Compare and Despair.

Television and magazines bombard us with images of so-called beauty ideals that look nothing like you or me. The motive? To keep us second-guessing our own worth. We see shot after shot of celebrities who are glorified when they are "perfect" and vilified when they "let themselves go." We're encouraged to judge these stars. And we do.

Comparison games create corrosive thought patterns, patterns that push us to talk negatively about ourselves and pit us against our fellow ladies. We all suffer the consequences.

Consider how many of us look at a photograph of a pretty woman—or, should I say, of a woman who fits with what society has dictated as pretty. First, we notice her beauty and appreciate it for its own sake. Then, about a half second later, that inner critic starts piping up: "I look nothing like her. Therefore, I'm hideous." I can almost hear the announcer right there alongside you: "Yes indeed, ladies. Another great afternoon ruined by a fun-filled round of Compare and Despair! Dedicated to keeping you in your place by knocking your spirit!"

I want off that not-so-merry-go-round. How about you?

We *are* society so, it is up to us to choose how we respond to what we see. The media and marketers will only change if we change our thinking and our behavior. Thank goodness, it's already starting to happen. For example, I applaud companies like Dove for their revolutionary Campaign for Real Beauty. Now is the perfect time to be your own beauty revolutionary, to stand up for what's yours and to act accordingly.

Now, don't get me wrong; *admiring* other women can be inspiring. As a kid, I idolized Marilyn Monroe and tried to emulate eighties supermodel Kim Alexis—both blondes with light eyes. Coincidence? Hardly. I find most women fixate on celebs who match their coloring, as if these stars are the ultimate remix of their own features. But guess what? If you were the famous one, those same people would be talking about *your* beauty.

After all, the actual definition of celebrity is "one who is celebrated." Want to be a celebrity? Start celebrating yourself! Decide that comparing and despairing is tedious and toxic, whether the standard you're applying is that of a fashion model or a woman at the gym. Recognize that there will *always* be someone more "this" and someone less "that." But the one with the most confidence wins every time. Resolve not to waste another minute keeping score.

You have far better ways to use that newfound time and energy.

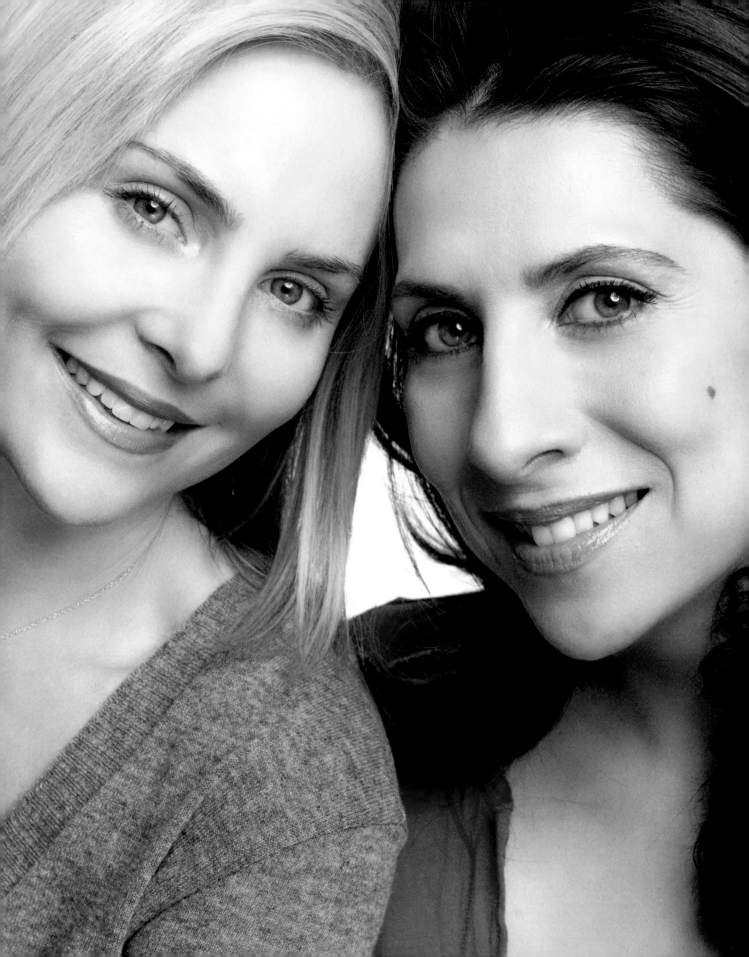

Revel in *Your* Fantastic Features

When I meet a woman for the first time, I automatically zoom in on her most compelling features and think of ways to enhance her unique beauty. It's just how my "expert" eye works. I hope to impart that same technique to you!

To start seeing with Carmindy Vision, I need your agreement on a couple of things. One: There is *no* set standard of feminine beauty. And two: Every woman is born blessed with something she can claim as beautiful . . .

- a large and powerful nose that is elegant and strong
- darkness under the eyes that creates a mysterious, sultry glance
- a crooked mouth that offers life and character to a smile
- a round face with large cheeks that looks warm and inviting
- a narrow face with a little chin that evokes a sweet charm

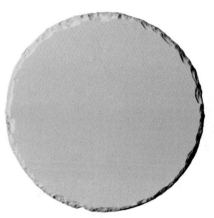

Excuse me while I enthuse. Lashes, brows, foreheads, cheeks, lips, skin! Such variety! So much to adore! Take a look! *Really* look at yourself and the women around you. Aren't we spectacular?

Case in point: my paternal grandmother. Grandma Hallie wasn't classically gorgeous, but to me she was the most beautiful woman ever because she took her best assets and worked the room with 'em. She had amazing skin and great lips, so she always rocked a red lipstick and wore silver bangles to play up her headliners. Outstanding.

Later in the book, we'll delve deeper into how to pinpoint your feature focus and enhance the best of what only you have to offer. Right now, I need your heartfelt, hardcore commitment to believing in your own beauty.

My expertise with lipsticks and shadows will fall flat without your full-on faith in *you*. But *with* it? Honey, you'll feel empowered, look incredible, and be unstoppable!

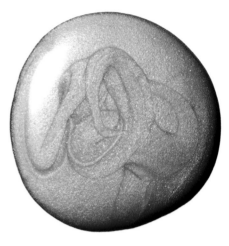

Embrace the Beauty Ritual

Many of us get excited at the thought of transforming our approach to beauty but stop short of doing it. Why? Because we've been told that pampering ourselves is selfish. Again, the negative voices start in. *Shouldn't you be spending that time on the kids? Or hubby? Or the boss? Anyone but you?*

The fact is, making time to enhance your natural beauty is your feminine privilege and can improve every aspect of your busy life. When you decide to put your best face forward, you start generating positive momentum and ride through the day on a wave of confidence. And when you're clearly confident, others believe in you, too. Believe it!

Embrace the power of the beauty ritual, and see what happens when you greet each day feeling relaxed, balanced, and at your best. Whether it's a bubble bath, a luxurious application of lotion, or a tender patting of powder on your nose, find a ritual that restores you, and do it to your heart's content.

We have history on our side here. The act of applying creams and cosmetics to benefit skin and spotlight features is an ancient, spiritual art form women have been performing for thousands of years. Check out the murals in King Tut's tomb. Those Egyptian ladies took their sweet time perfecting their kohl-black eyes. Why shouldn't you take a few minutes in the morning to nurture your own beauty?

Consider your beauty ritual as the one steadfast opportunity you have to breathe deeply, rid yourself of negative thoughts, and honor your loveliness. You need never apologize for making yourself a priority, nor for taking womanly pleasure in it.

And guess what? When you let go of negativity and take a positive, playful attitude toward beauty, you'll lighten your load and free up a lot of headspace and heart space to be more giving to others. And you'll be an even better mom, wife, friend, or colleague because you'll have started the day with a strong foundation of feeling good about yourself. Nothing selfish about it!

Change the Game and Win Every Time

I've asked you to change the way you think, to tell the naysayers to buzz off and to focus on your assets. Simply put, to change for the better. But let's face it: change of any kind can be scary.

All fear boils down to the fear of the unknown. We hold on to negative thoughts and counterproductive habits if for no other reason than we're used to them. They've hung around *for years.* Good old, boring status quo. To that I say *heave-ho*!

Be brave enough to live life beautifully. You may not have traveled this road before; you may not know where it's going. But trust me, it leads to a fascinating new place filled with opportunities, adventures, and unimaginable satisfaction.

Some of you might hold back your best for fear of standing out in the crowd. You might confuse confidence with arrogance. To that I must ask, why are you so comfortable underplaying yourself? How is settling for less serving anyone?

When you tune in to what's special about you, you turn on an inner light that brightens the way for everyone you encounter. When you switch your focus to the positive, you feel energized and kind, creating a presence that is peaceful and comforting to others.

Your feeling good and looking it radiates goodness out into the world. Beauty is magical. It's powerful. And it only attracts more of the good stuff we want to come into the lives we share. Paying attention to beauty isn't narcissistic, it's downright humanitarian!

Albert Einstein once said, "The definition of insanity is doing the same thing over and over again and expecting different results." Clearly, you picked up this book to achieve something different for yourself, not only for your looks but also for your life. So how about we end the insanity?

If we're going to be obsessed, let's be obsessed with being positive. Let's focus our energies on playing up our natural beauty and appreciating the unique gifts of everyone around us. Let's expect different results; let's expect the best!

You know, the *only* thing separating the dreamers from the achievers is action. Getting positively beautiful is an easy way to initiate change. Just take that first step, and keep on going.

It's your life, sugar. Make it *gorgeous!*

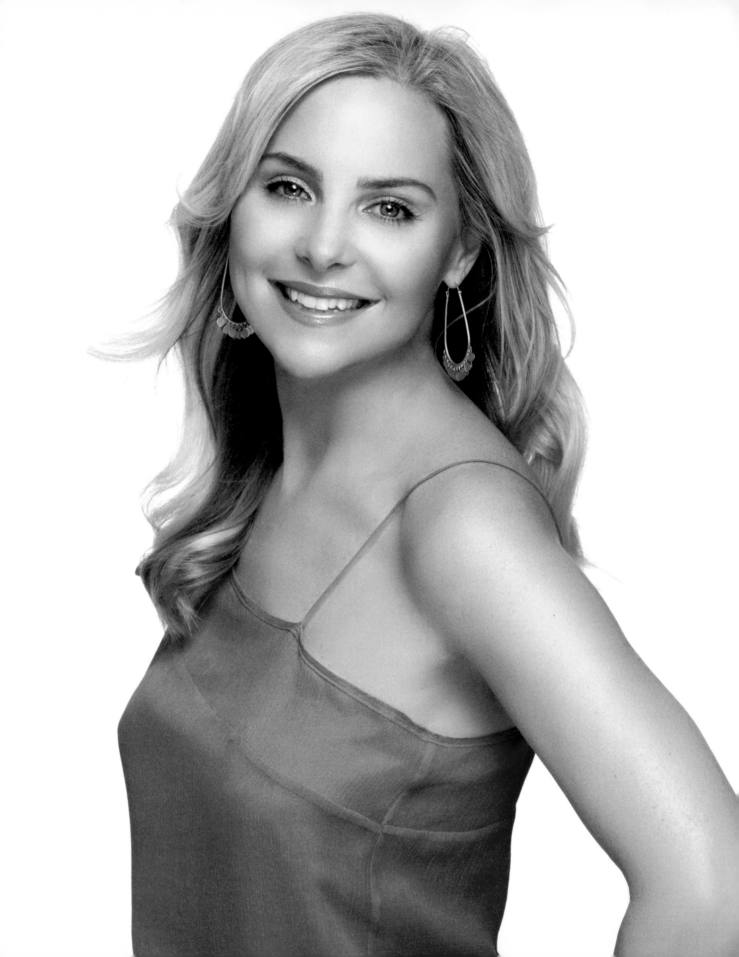

carmindy's beauty journey

I wasn't always as confident as I am now. It's been a process. And now that I think about it, it's been about coming into my own by coming full circle.

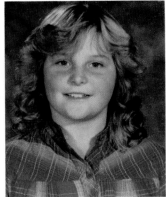

Me at age 11

When I was a little girl, I always thought I was special and that I was destined to have a really amazing life. My parents were loving and rock-solid supportive. Up until the fourth grade, I never looked at myself as anything but a shining light of happiness.

But when I was about ten or eleven, all that confidence and self-esteem flew out the window when kids started hurling cruel remarks at me. I had never looked at myself in a negative way until other kids pointed out my "failings."

I was chubby, wore braces, had a bad eighties perm, and freckles that I should have been loving but was instead being teased about. Classmates called me "basketball head." They snickered about my non-designer clothing. Their taunts of "thunder thighs, fat butt" echoed in my head.

I remember one day in art class, we traced our silhouettes onto construction paper and hung them up for fellow students to identify. One kid said, "Oh, you can tell which one Carmindy is—the one with the double chin." That comment stayed with me *for years*.

When junior high hit, I started playing with makeup—or, should I say, piling it on. I slathered on foundation to cover my freckles. I smudged loads of brown powder into my cheeks in an attempt to contour away the "basketball" roundness. And eyes? I'm surprised I could lift my lids! Not only did I overcompensate, I did a poor job of it.

Like many women, I let others' opinions shape how I felt about my looks.

I remember saving up for a trip to a fancy hair salon. When I sat in that chair, the stylist told me I had a *huge* forehead and should always wear bangs. So I followed his orders for fear of blinding people with my enormous dome.

While I was busy trying to disguise my flaws, I was doing something else entirely: erasing my true self and extinguishing that bright, shiny light I used to feel as that "star" of a little girl.

But when I started doing makeup professionally, learning about techniques and seeing features differently, I began finding beauty in so many people. Including me.

There wasn't one *aha* moment. But I started questioning those old criticisms. *What were those nasty people talking about? Why was I giving them any of my energy? Why was I still hearing their voices?*

I decided to shut them up and start listening to my inner voice instead. A round face is just as lovely as a narrow one; foreheads big or small mean nothing in terms of self-worth. I began embracing myself by focusing on the positive. Buh-bye, makeup mask!

At the mirror, my mantra was no longer, *Ugh, these cheeks.* It became, *Hey gorgeous, look at those great eyes and fantastic smile.* Was it easy to do? Nope. But I was determined to change my life, one positive thought at a time.

And guess what? It totally changed everything.

I retrained my brain beyond how I thought about my looks. I used every spare moment to envision feeling happy and confident and energized. If I caught myself being self-critical, I'd put on the brakes and force myself to say something kind and inspiring.

During this transformation, I went a little overboard in the other direction: I stopped wearing makeup altogether. Somehow I needed to face the world with a naked face in order to re-create my self-image. Step-by-step, I learned new makeup techniques and used myself as a guinea pig. If I tried something out and it looked like a mask, I would take it off and not use it on anybody else.

I learned how to polish my own natural beauty and did the same with my clients. I noticed that if I simply played up their best features—using only the right products in the right places—women sparkled more than if I gave them the full-on application.

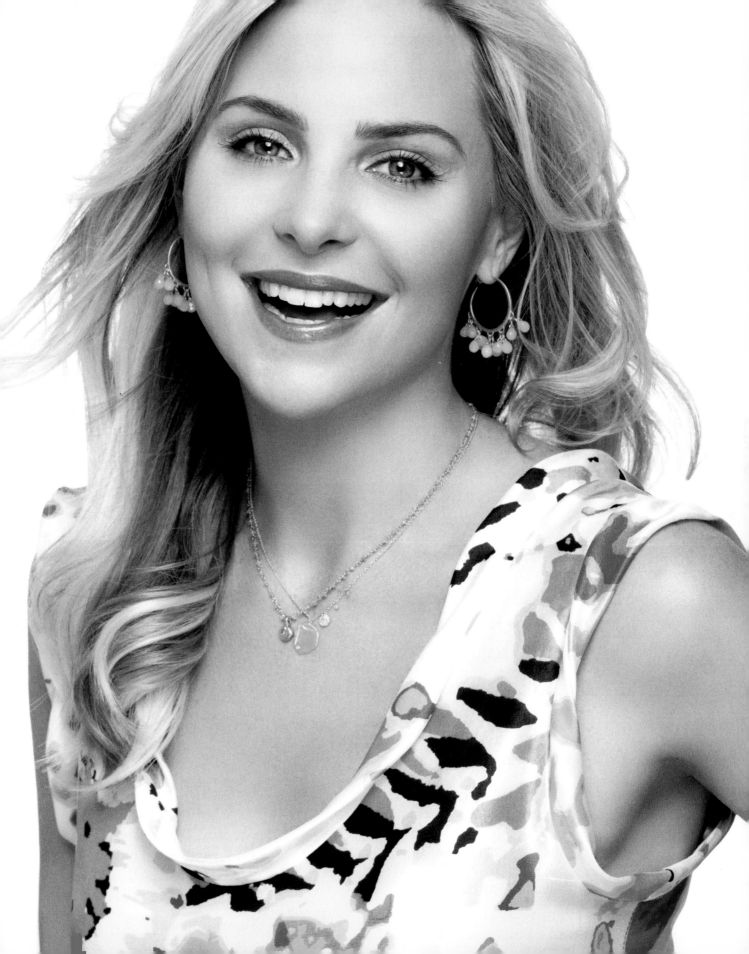

You might think a complete makeover with a totally new face painted on would be a wonderful surprise. I'm here to tell you it isn't true. You might say "wow," but you wouldn't sparkle; you'd be startled because you wouldn't recognize yourself.

But when you enhance your unique assets, you delight in seeing your best self, the one you always knew was there. The true, beautiful you.

I've seen it a thousand times! Beauty radiates with a hundred times the oomph when a woman powers up her potential and puts her best features forward. *Hey world, this is me! To the* n*th degree!*

Confidence exudes beauty; insecurity undercuts it. I've worked with models who were considered to be

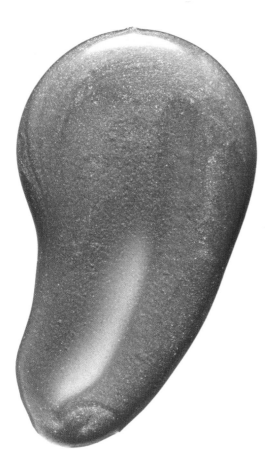

the feminine ideal yet felt horrible about their appearance. They obsessed over the smallest flaw, ignoring their blessings. And you know what? I wouldn't trade faces with any of 'em. Self-hatred isn't pretty.

Today I prefer to treasure what I have instead of wasting time and energy on playing comparison games. I like to say *I polish what I own.* I don't try to change it, re-create it, or conjure it up with hocus-pocus trickery. I just take really, really good care of myself—emotionally and physically—and walk out the door every day feeling great.

Someone once asked me, "When do you feel most beautiful?" I told her it happens every day, twice a day. First, when I step out of the shower feeling fresh and clean and take a moment to slather on some creamy lotion. And second, when I first step onto the sidewalk, working my 5-minute face. I know I've enhanced my natural beauty with a little foundation, highlighter, cheek and lip color, and definition around the eyes. I just feel like I've taken care of me and can now let the day bring me its challenges and triumphs. I'm ready for anything!

MY PAMPERING RITUAL

Each morning, I exfoliate my face by lightly scrubbing it with plain white sugar, a great technique and money saver. Good thing, too, because next I dip into my big splurge: Crème de la Mer moisturizer. It's my little pamperng treat.

Even how I apply it is ritualized. I tap my fingers in the jar, then tap the formula all over my face in little dots. With my ring fingers (the gentlest ones!), I just blend it in using small, circular movements—a mini facial massage. Delish.

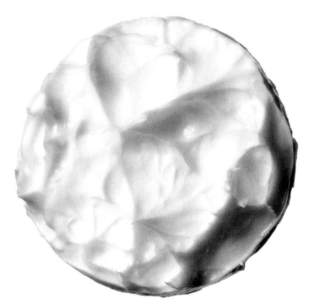

Getting to this place of peaceful confidence wasn't easy, but it was as simple as deciding to take one step in that direction. Then the next one. And another. It's an *incredibly* freeing journey I hope you'll take and make your own.

So come on! Dump that boring, negative tape filled with those discouraging voices of people who don't mean a thing to you today. And instead, embrace the best parts of you, nurturing your gifts so they grow and expand to arenas far beyond the mirror.

When you change your focus to the positive, you turn on a certain light and energy that attracts all the good stuff.

And oh honey, how you'll shine!

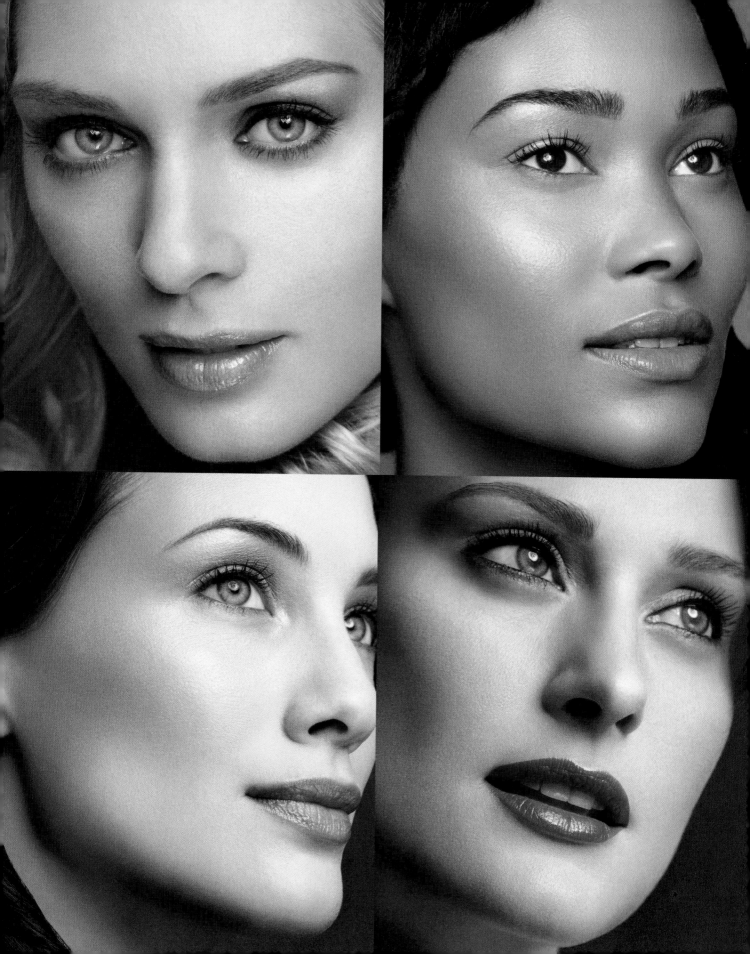

To be irreplaceable, one must always be different.
—COCO CHANEL

chapter three find your feature focus

Style icon Coco Chanel knew it, and so do you: Unique is chic.

The great news? Every woman's face offers a unique blend of features and expressiveness. So every woman—(*me?* Yes, you!)—has the potential to be irreplaceably lovely. The key? Celebrating your best assets and enhancing them to the hilt!

Discovering your best features and learning how to highlight them is not only fun but liberating. When you start focusing on only the good, you gradually get rid of the destructive self-talk that's been binding up your mind and sapping your energy. Practicing a positive beauty attitude will brighten both your face and your spirit. Guaranteed.

Boost Your Self-Confidence

Numero uno: Replace your old flaw fixations with a new focus on your best features.

Now, I hear you. *Easier said than done.* But remember dear Einstein from chapter one. If you want to feel different and are serious about looking your best, some serious reprogramming is in order. Commit to thinking differently about your beauty. Start now.

Close your eyes and visualize your face. Shut down any negative comments at the first peep, and concentrate instead on one thing you've always liked about your looks. Is it those dimples when you smile? Those lashes that flare out at the corners? The bowlike fullness of those lips? Only you know the answer.

Next, step up to the mirror and really take in how wonderful that attribute is. *Gorgeous and mine!*

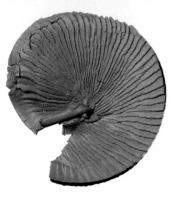

See with Carmindy Vision

Next, look away for a second and then look back quickly for what I call a flash glance of Carmindy Vision. Did you spot something else that's extraordinary? Look again. You know it's there, and so do I. Voilà! You've found your feature focus. Maybe it's one amazing asset or several strengths. The important thing is that you're focusing on what's fabulous, and you're on your way!

Now, if you tend to be the "Tough on Myself Champion of the World" and still can't see with Carmindy Vision, don't just stand there. Get a second opinion! Ask a loving and trusted family member, "What do you like best about my face?" or ask your best girlfriend to close her eyes and imagine your face. Then ask, "What do you think of first? What makes my face special?" Chances are, people around you have long admired something special about your beauty. Many may have complimented you on it, and you either didn't hear it or didn't want to believe it. Instead of being tough on yourself, be tough on negativity. Pay attention to the positive observations of others and *believe them*.

Retrain Your Brain with Mirror Mantras

Don't waste yourself in rejection, nor bark against the bad, but chant in the beauty of the good. —RALPH WALDO EMERSON

Remember this line from *Snow White and the Seven Dwarfs? Mirror, mirror on the wall, who's the fairest of them all?* To get positively beautiful, you must play fair with your looks!

You've already made great strides in the right direction by finding your feature focus. Keep that momentum going by starting each day with a mirror mantra.

A mirror mantra is an uplifting statement you say to yourself while looking in the mirror. There's no better face-lift in the world than speaking positively about your beauty.

In an instant, you can simply change your thoughts, speak caring words, and channel your whole spirit toward appreciation. And that looks so good on you!

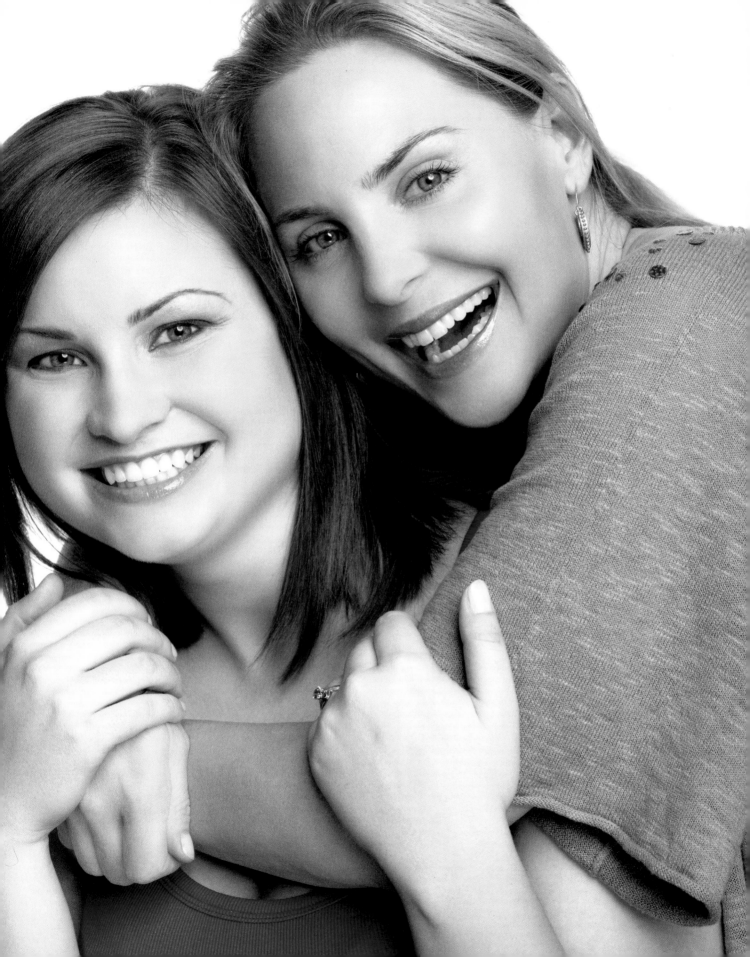

Remember what I said about thoughts and words being powerful? What's incredible about beauty affirmations is that they work even if you don't fully believe what you're saying at first.

It's a matter of physics. What? Science in a beauty book? Go with me on this . . .

Your thoughts are bursts of molecular energy speeding through your brain. That energy is as real and measurable as that of sunlight or a waterfall. When you force yourself to think and say something positive, your brain fires on its positive pistons. Your little molecules vibrate on the positive setting. Because all energies attract other energies of the same sort, your brain starts looking for more positive vibes. You literally start to see and experience more positive stuff in your world and in yourself. Kinda freaky, right? Also miraculous and true!

Bottom line, you can retrain your brain to see yourself and everything else more beautifully. What a gift that is.

Good Mornin', Sunshine!

Each morning, fire up your good vibrations with a mirror mantra. You've already pinpointed your favorite features. Now praise 'em loud and proud. Here are a few examples to get you rolling . . .

My skin is creamy and dreamy.
What amazing cheekbones I have!
My eyes look so sparkling and cheerful.

Come on, really let me hear ya! Sing it as a song. Turn it into a rhyme. It doesn't matter *how* you do it as long as you commit yourself to *doing it.* Take delight in the moment, and take no notice of anyone who might mock your efforts. Do you feel foolish? Stop and ask yourself, "Isn't it more foolish to stay trapped in insecurities and be attracting negative energy to my day?" Uh-huh!

Do enough of these mirror mantras, and pretty soon you'll discover that your negative self-talk has stopped. You'll feel a newfound appreciation not only for your individual beauty but for the beauty of others. Your positive brain will be in control, and you'll charge forward with confidence—the most attractive asset of all.

Rx for Mirror-of-Doom Moments

We all have them: those days when we're feeling exhausted, over-whelmed, or just plain out of sorts, those moments when the mirror adds fuel to the flames of negativity. (It happens to me in airplane lavatories. The worst!)

What to do when the mirror-of-doom strikes?

Don't stare. Don't drag out the cosmetics and start shoveling on every product under the sun. Don't give the blahs any energy.

Do be a good mother to yourself. When you've had a tough day or are not feeling quite so fabulous, give yourself a break. Instead of standing there and hating yourself, remember that the moment you feed a negative cycle of criticism by focusing on what's so clearly very, very wrong with you, you've let the bad vibes take over—and they are greedy little buggers! Instead, pamper your pucker with a little lip balm and *move on.*

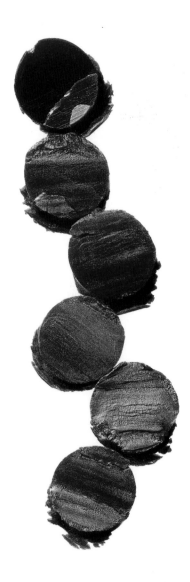

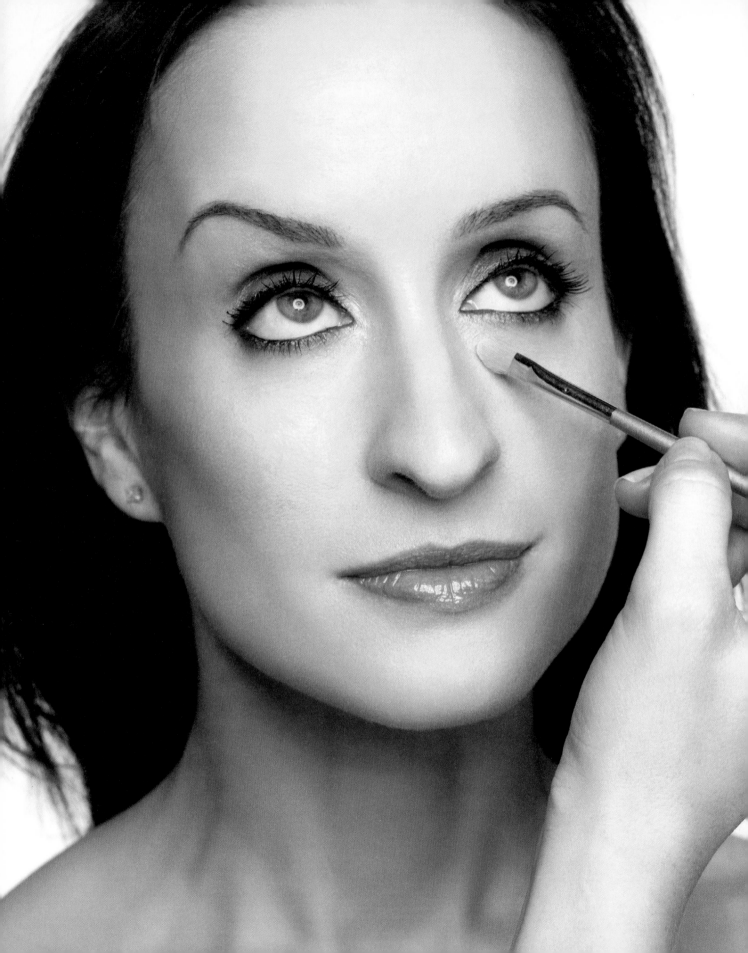

There are flowers everywhere, for those who bother to look.

—HENRI MATISSE

chapter four
use makeup to illuminate your beauty

Many experts say that makeup is best understood as the art of creating an illusion.

They advise us to trick the eye into seeing what is not true. Their techniques emphasize contouring a face to conform to a certain beauty standard and they push flaw-concealment as priority one.

Well, not here. Not me. No way. Because your beauty is no illusion!

Readers of *The 5-Minute Face* will recall how my inspiration to become a makeup artist came from watching my mother paint her canvases with watercolors. She used gentle brushstrokes, swirled in soft washes of color, and played with light to draw the eye to what was wonderful about her subject.

Ladies, today our subject is you. And Mom's modus operandi still applies. (Thanks, Mom!)

Since reading the last chapter, I hope you've already started seeing your features in new ways and found a favorite or three. What you're about to learn is how to light up your best features by using the right products in the right places. Step-by-step, I'll show you how to illuminate your natural assets so your unique loveliness shines through. All you. All true. *Positively beautiful.*

As you explore each of the following chapters, set your attitude on playful adventure. You may consider your eyes your best feature, but there's every reason to try new ways to showcase your lips, cheeks, or skin. Let your spirit be your guide. Is today a sexy-lips day or a bronzed-cheek day? Does tonight call for a moody eye or an elegantly minimalist look? Remember, it's makeup. There are no goofs you can't wash off, so why not go for it?

Now let's have some fun getting your gorgeousness on!

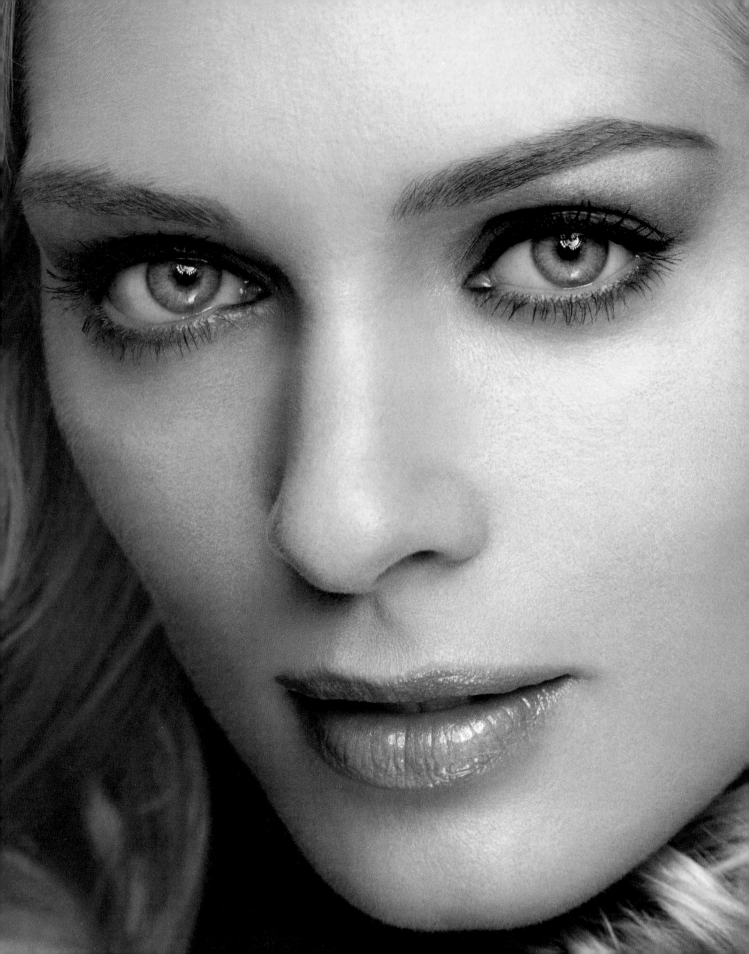

The face is the mirror of the mind, and eyes without

speaking confess the secrets of the heart.

—SAINT JEROME

chapter five the eyes have it

Connection. Soulfulness. Enchantment. Our eyes speak volumes without making a sound. So, what have yours been saying lately? By this point in our little voyage together, I hope it's a whole lotta sweet somethings!

Eyes are a fantastic feature to focus on as you shift your beauty thinking. Every color, every shape, at every age—eyes have an irresistible allure all their own. By refining your approach to eye makeup, you can supercharge your whole face. Believe it!

Electrify Those Irises

The most frequently asked question I hear is, "How do I make my eyes stand out?"

"Opposites attract" is my motto when enhancing eyes to look vividly alive. By choosing shadows, liners, and mascaras that contrast with your eye color, you turn up the voltage of your irises for an electrifying beauty. Whether your peepers are blue, green, brown, or hazel, using opposing makeup colors will always make them "pop."

Now remember, there are no hard-and-fast rules; the following are only suggestions to help you sensationalize your eyes. Play with this "opposites attract" idea, and pay attention to the compliments sure to follow!

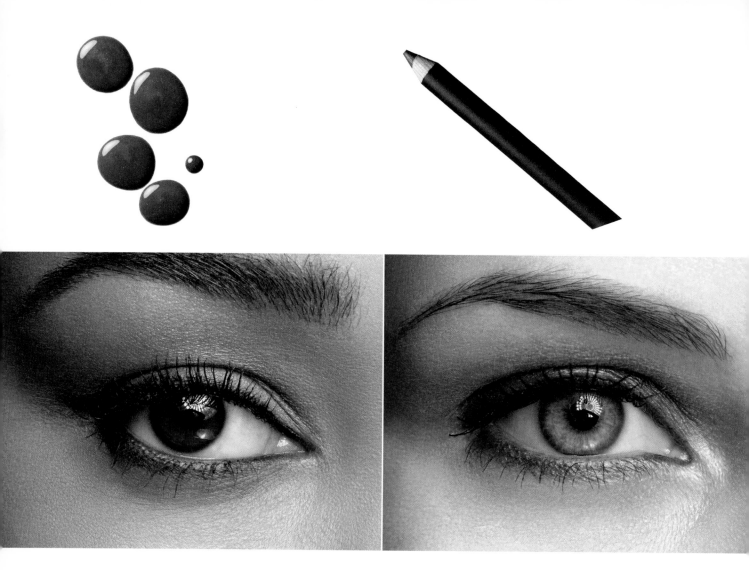

BROWN EYES

Play with deep shades of navy and sapphire smudged into the lash line for a subtle edge that is alluring but not over-the-top. When using blue eyeliner, follow with neutral lid colors like soft shimmering browns for a modern look.

Brown-eyed girls can also have fun with shades of green. Experiment with forest and emerald to discover what really sparkles on you.

BLUE EYES

Smudge on shades of chocolate brown, taupe, or bronze to make the blue really come alive. Blue shadows compete with your natural color, so play to the positive by skipping blue hues.

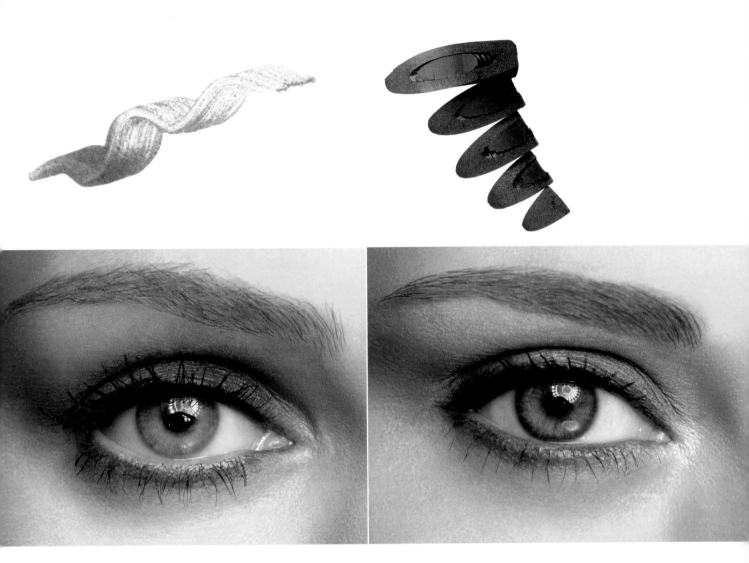

GREEN EYES

Try eyeliners or shadows in eggplant, purple,
burgundy, lavender, or amethyst. The contrast of
colors will give you the sexiest emerald stare.

HAZEL EYES

Hazel eyes look incredible when paired with green shadow.
My personal favorite is a sparkling forest green applied
across the lid and under the lash line. This shade deepens
the brown tones while bringing up the green.

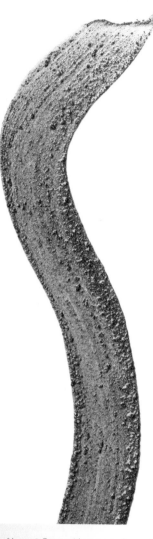

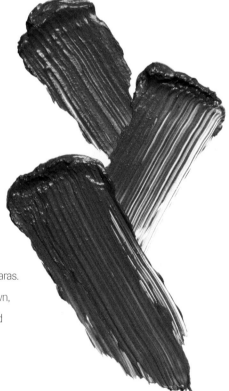

When playing up your gorgeous eyes, remember to balance your total look by toning down lip color so the eyes are the star of the show.

Feeling faint of heart? Start with a neutral eye shadow and add an "opposites attract" liner shade on the underside of the upper lash line for a slight hint of color.

Not a huge fan of eye shadow? Check out tinted mascaras. Look for dark hues of deep green, navy blue, teak brown, or rich plum. (Anything lighter will be distracting instead of alluring.)

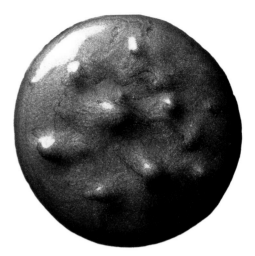

Liquid Eyeliner

We ooh and ahh over eyes perfectly defined with liquid liner, yet most of us shy away from trying it out ourselves. Shake off the intimidation, ladies! *Every* woman can wear liquid liner to create an enchanting, entrancing glance.

Today's liquid liner formulas go on smooth and keep flaking at bay, and many are waterproof for lasting wear. Black is the classic color choice but far from the only option. For added zing, try teal, eggplant, shimmering brown, silver, or bronze. Look for liners featuring a small, tapered brush and a shorter handle—they're much easier to control than the longer, skinny ones.

Ready to give liquid liner a go? Fantastic. Here's my foolproof technique: get out your magnifying mirror, get up close, and give yourself a wink!

- The secret to applying liquid liner like a pro is not trying to sweep on a perfect line all at once. Begin applying liquid liner as close to the roots of the lashes as possible, starting at the inside corner of the eyes. In little connecting dashes, work your way toward the outer corners, and finish with a little sweep up at the ends. This little wing lifts the eyes and opens them up.
- Personally, I never apply liquid liner under the lower lash line; it looks too harsh. For subtle under-eye definition, sweep on a touch of powdered shadow instead by using an angle brush. I like to finish my liquid liner look with neutral shadows on the lid and crease.
- If you have a very shaky hand or are a newbie to liquid liners, try drawing the line with a pencil liner first, then trace over it with liquid liner.
- Don't fret if the line isn't perfect. Simply dip a small-tipped concealer brush into a little foundation, and use it as a perfecting eraser. No worries!

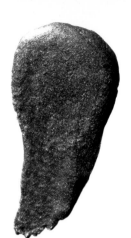

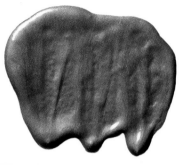

Have blonde eyelash roots you just can't reach with mascara? Paint them with black liquid eyeliner.

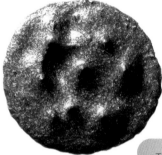

Use liquid eyeliner to hide the seam on false lashes.

Try dipping an angle brush into liquid liner and sweeping it across the eye for a slightly thicker, more controlled line.

Here are a few tailored tips for liquid liner loveliness. If you have . . .

SMALLER EYES — keep the line thin and close to the lashes

BIGGER EYES — draw on a thicker line

DEEP-SET EYES — try your "opposites attract" shade instead of black or brown to brighten the area

ALMOND EYES — extend the line to a subtle wing at each end

HOODED EYES — always choose a waterproof formula; keep liner close to the roots of the lashes; once applied, keep looking down until the liner is completely dry to prevent smudging

WIDE-SET EYES — start lining the eyes a bit thicker on the inside corners and then thin the line as you work your way toward the ends; no wings, please!

CLOSE-SET EYES — start the line slightly past the midpoint of the upper lids; work outward and wing out at the ends

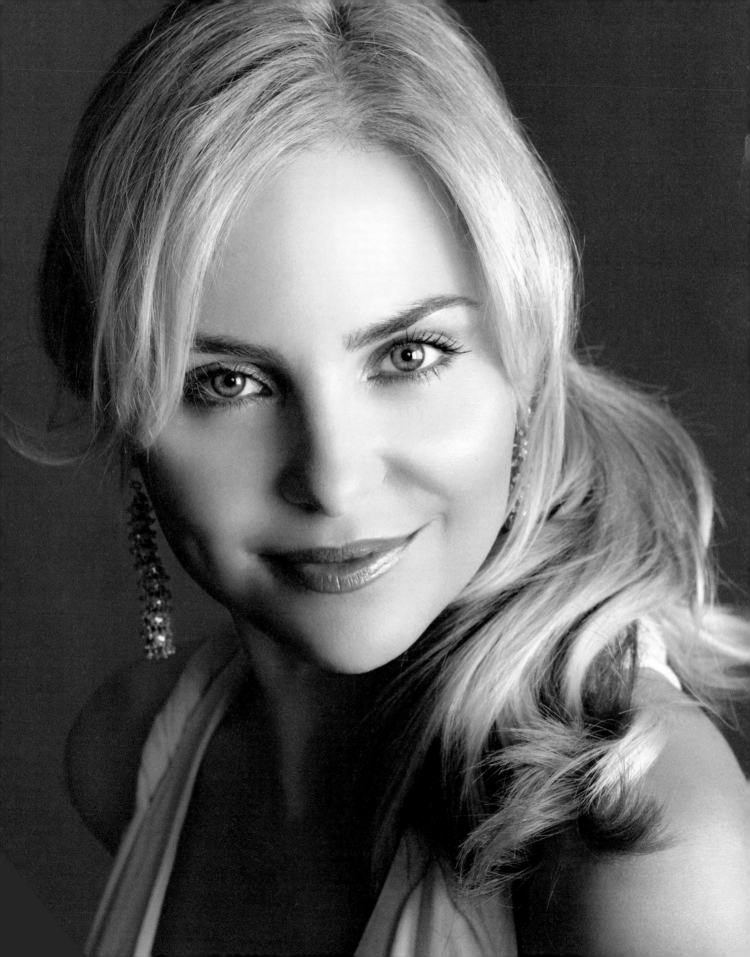

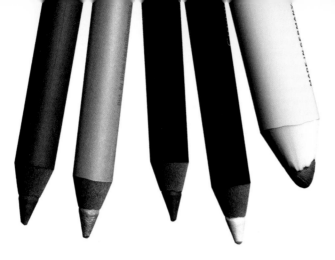

For a dramatic, extra-thick lash line, apply black eyeliner on the upper inside rim of the eye at the bottom base of the lashes.

Pencil Eyeliner

Pencil eyeliners offer a more natural approach to eye definition and are supereasy to apply. Whether you choose a smudgy rock-n-roll look or a fine, barely there line, your eyes will command attention.

Look for pencils that glide on smooth and don't pull or tug the delicate eye area. I like gel liners that slick on seamlessly and stay put all day. For women with hooded lids or oily skin, a waterproof formula will last for hours without smudges. To ensure the most precise application, always sharpen the pencil first.

- Start by tilting your head up so you are looking down your nose into the mirror. (While you're at it, say *hello, sassy!*) From this position, you can see your entire lid.
- Gently pull your eyelid taut with your ring finger at the outer corner of the eye and begin drawing the pencil along the lash line, wiggling color into the roots as you go. Now shade in any visible skin between the liner and the lashes. Lovely!
- To achieve an even softer effect, trace over the liner with an angle brush that has been dipped into a little powder eye shadow.
- For superdrama, try layering liner. I like to line the eyes with a dark color, like black or deep chocolate brown. Then I place a lighter shade, like blue or burgundy, right above the dark liner for a rich, thick lash line look.
- Feeling a touch unsteady? Breathe! Then feather on light strokes of pencil and blend 'em together with a cotton swab or an angle brush for a soft, natural-looking finish.

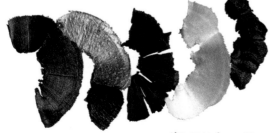

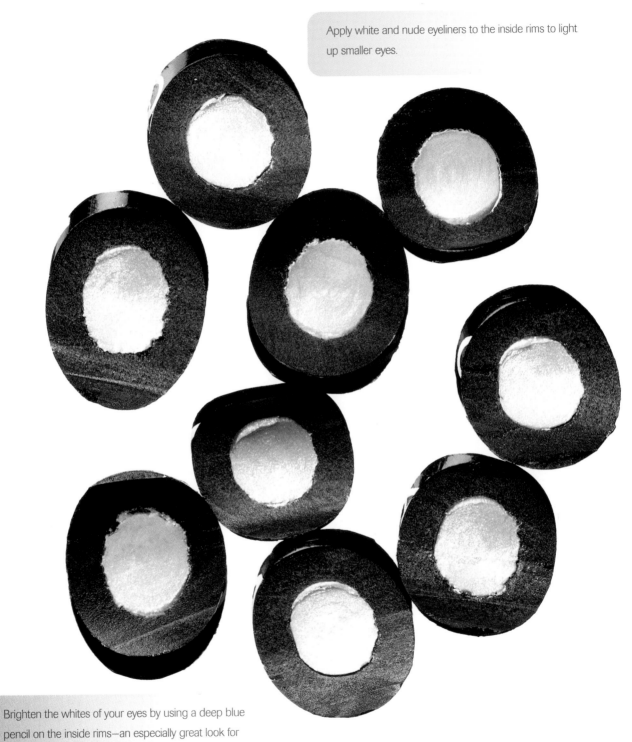

Apply white and nude eyeliners to the inside rims to light up smaller eyes.

Brighten the whites of your eyes by using a deep blue pencil on the inside rims—an especially great look for women with darker skin.

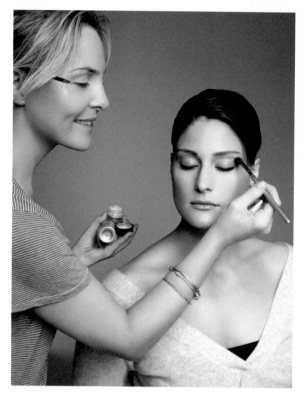

Choose dark liners that contain shimmer for extra sparkle.

Eye Shadow

Eye shadows come in so many colors and formulas; the sky's the limit for playful possibilities. Light layers of different tones can make your eyes look alluring, mysterious, sexy, flirty, or downright fabulous. Use eye shadows to enhance the natural shape of your eyes, not reinvent it. Think use, not abuse!

You always want at least three shades to experiment with: the highlight shadow, the midtone shadow, and the contour shadow.

HIGHLIGHT SHADOW

The highlight shadow is the key to my whole "Carmindy look." I love highlighting because it turns the light around your eyes on high. You instantly glow and look luminous.

Highlighter shades include a pale palette of white; champagne; vanilla; pearled pink; and light, iridescent, or sunset gold. Choose matte or pearl shades for mature skin and shimmer for younger skin.

Play with highlight eye shadow on areas to which you want to draw attention. Try a dab on the center of the lid. Sweep it under the brow for a high-arch look. Place it on the inside corners for a sparkling, eye-opening effect. Amazing!

Highlighting works so well, you can skip the other two shades when you want a quick, out-the-door look. By virtue of its light color, your bare eyelid appears darker in contrast, as if you're already wearing shadow on the lid.

Clearly, highlighter is the superstar of shadows, but its two costars provide bountiful options to change up your look to suit any occasion.

Mirror Mantra
I love having two different-colored eyes, one brown and one hazel. They both change color according to what I am wearing!
Karen, 43, Louisville, KY

MIDTONE SHADOW

Your midtone shadow is used to create a subtle enhancement to the shape of the eye. Choose a shade just slightly darker than your natural skin tone, no matter what the color. Darker-skinned ladies, go deep; paler women, stay in medium tones. When blended into the right spots, your midtone shadow can create more depth or more mystery. Most of the time, it adds an appealing hue to lids.

CONTOUR SHADOW

Finally, your darker contour shadow creates drama, definition, and intensity. Stay in the same family of colors as your midtone; just go deeper. Place this darkest shadow at the outer corner of the eye or in the crease, or use it as a soft liner.

Gilded goodness: Try a dot of silver or gold at the inner corners or on the center of the lid for a glittery good time.

Color play: If you want to try a blue, green, purple, or burgundy shadow, don't cover the whole eye area. Pinpoint one area, like the lash line or the lid, to avoid looking overdone.

For softer definition, use an angle brush to sweep on dark eye shadow as a liner, or use your favorite shadow as a cake liner by wetting the brush.

Mascara

Mascara opens up the eyes to make them look their most fluttery fabulous. If you're blessed with long, lush lashes, mascara is the magic tool to glorify them. If you have a finer fringe of lashes, mascara helps make the most of every single one. Consider it a beauty staple and an eye-look plus for every occasion.

Cosmetics companies recognize mascara's appeal and have introduced all sorts of brushes, combs, paints, polymers, primers, lengtheners, thickeners, and more. Check out some of the innovations, and find your fave. To skip smudginess, try waterproof formulas or the new "tube" technology mascaras. Those babies last all day without a single smear.

If you use an eyelash curler, always do so *before* applying mascara. Crimping after mascara causes breakage—not what we're after here!

One other no-no: don't pump the wand in and out of the tube. This is as pointless as shaking a Polaroid. The action dries out the mascara and often loads too much onto the brush—a one-way ticket to Goopyville.

Lash out by applying one easy sweep of highlight across the entire lid, and double dose your lashes with black mascara on top and bottom. Drama delish!

Hold a plastic spoon under the lower lash line while applying mascara. Smudges wind up on the spoon, not on your skin. Genius!

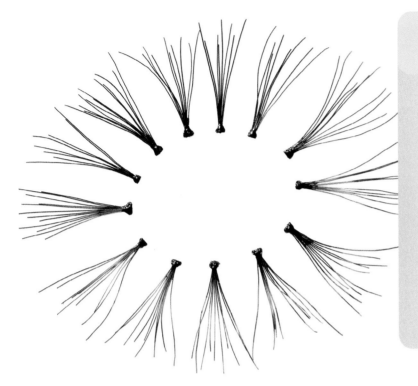

To create a natural look, sweep on one easy coat, starting with the brush at the base of the lashes and using a zigzagging motion up to the tips. For extra drama, reapply a second coat or concentrate another application only at the outer corners. When it's lower-lash time, first lightly wipe off the wand with a paper towel and then hold the brush vertically, waving it back and forth. Stupendous!

I prefer smaller mascara wands, as they offer more control and get to the hard-to-reach lashes. Keep a good lash comb on hand to separate any clumpies. For smudges, use a cotton swab or concealer brush dipped into foundation for a quick cleanup.

For ladies with thick lashes (you lucky bunch), try lining the lash line with golden bronze eyeliner or powdered eye shadow. Comb on black mascara and—curtain up—it's showtime!

For women with fine lashes, fire up the ka-pow by dotting dark eyeliner pencil in between each lash to bring out their full potential.

Classic Eye Looks

Fashions come and go, but these universal techniques enhance every lady's eyes and are always in style.

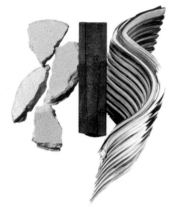

ON THE GO

For a quick-n-easy day look, apply highlight shadow under the brows and on the inside corners of the eyes. Next, lightly smudge pencil liner along the top lash lines and follow with black mascara on the top lashes only. Stopwatch says: mere seconds!

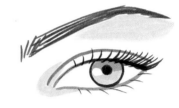

● Highlight

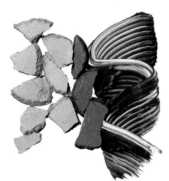

DAY TO NIGHT

For an eye that's ready for day or evening, lightly line the upper lash line with a pencil. Next, sweep a midtone shadow on the lid, and with an angle brush, smudge it under the lower lash line. Then brush a contour shadow in the crease and a highlight shade under the brow. Finish with mascara, and you're gorgeously good to go.

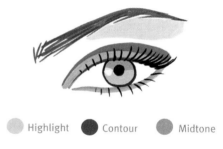

● Highlight   ● Contour   ● Midtone

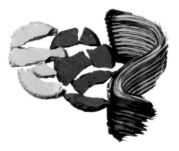

SULTRY AND SMOKY

Want a fast and foolproof smoky eye? Sweep a dark-hued contour eye shadow across the lid and under the lower lashes. Apply a midtone shade in the crease. Follow with a highlight shade under the brow and on the inside corners of the eyes. Polish off the look with black mascara, top and bottom, and you're ready for a great night out.

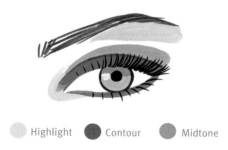

● Highlight   ● Contour   ● Midtone

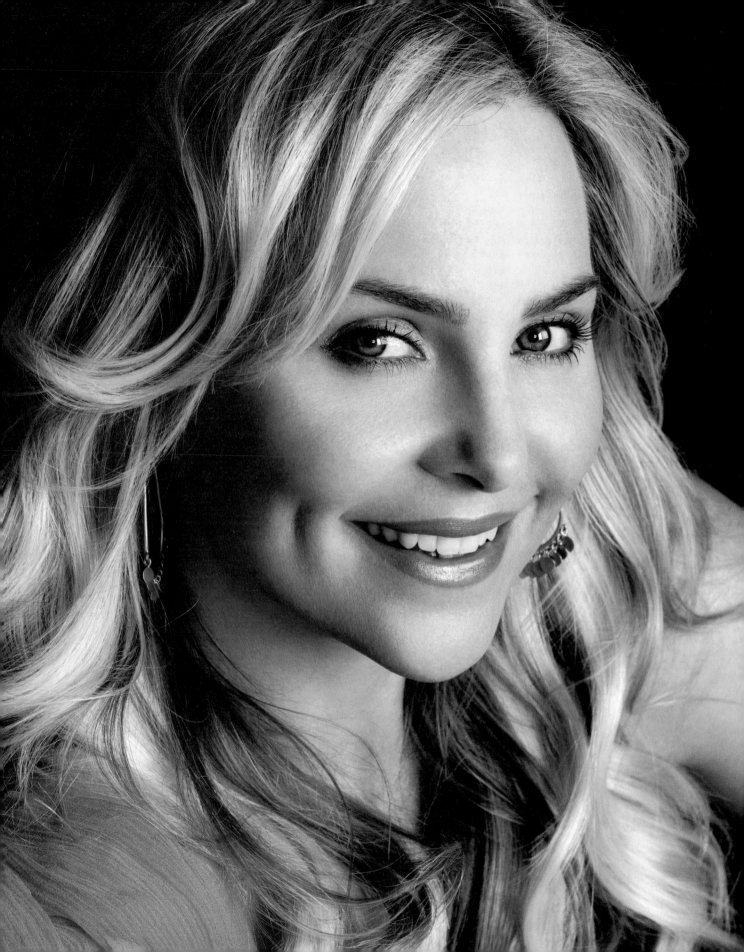

Custom Eye Looks

Seeing your individuality as a giftno is the key to getting positively beautiful. See how brightly you can shine when you experiment with an eye look customized to your unique assets.

SMALL EYES

To play up your petite, pretty peepers, the secret is to not go overboard with dark eye shadows.

1. Start by highlighting the entire lid with a light, shimmering shadow and blending it in so just a glow shows.
2. Next, sweep a midtone eye shadow into the crease.
3. Apply a small line of dark eyeliner across the outer half of the lid, as close to the roots of the upper lashes as possible (avoid a thick, heavy line on the upper lid).
4. Apply a midtone eye shadow (the same color as in the crease) under the lower lash line using an angle brush, starting in the center of the lower lid and moving outward. Then smudge to soften the effect.
5. Finish with mascara on the top and bottom lashes.

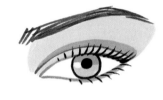

Highlight   Midtone

BIG EYES

If you have doll-like, beautiful eyes, enhance them with smoky eye shadows and lots of mascara.

1. Start by lining the upper and lower lash line with eyeliner in a deep shade.
2. Next, sweep a dark contour eye shadow color across the entire lid and under the lower lash line.
3. Follow with a midtone shade in the crease, and end with a highlight shade under the brow.
4. Apply a healthy dose of mascara on the top lashes only.

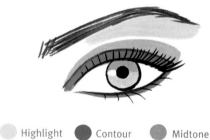

Highlight   Contour   Midtone

Mirror Mantra
I love the single freckle under my left eye. It used to bother me, but now I think of it as a beauty mark highlighting my strongest feature! Jessica, 23, Ottawa, ON

DEEP-SET EYES

For ladies with sexy, deep-set eyes, make them even more alluring by highlighting the lid and allowing the natural deep crease to stand out.

1. Start by sweeping a highlight shade with a hint of shimmer across the entire lid, from the lash line to the crease.

2. Next, apply a midtone eye shadow just above, not in, the crease.

3. Apply eyeliner across the upper lash line and use an angle brush to sweep a dark shadow in the same hue as the liner under the lower lash line.

4. Follow with mascara on the top and bottom lashes.

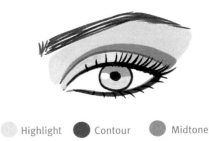

○ Highlight ● Contour ● Midtone

ALMOND EYES

An almond-eyed gal can showcase this fabulous feature by slightly exaggerating the sultry shape.

1. Try lining the upper lash line with dark liner and extending it out and up in a little wing.

2. Next, apply highlight shadow under the brow and on the inside corners of the eyes.

3. Sweep on a midtone eye shadow across the lid, from the lash line to the crease.

4. Follow with a darker contour shadow in the crease, and use an angle brush to smudge it under the lower lash line.

5. Apply one coat of mascara to all the lashes, then follow with a second layer just at the outer corners of the upper lashes.

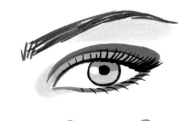

○ Highlight ● Contour ● Midtone

HOODED EYES

Hooded eyes can look enchantingly exotic. Increase your mysteriousness by applying a soft blend of shadows.

1. Start by applying highlight shadow under the brow and on the inside corners of the eyes.

2. Next, sweep a midtone shadow across the lid, from the lash line to slightly above the crease. The best way to find the crease is to gently push the eye shadow brush into the lid; your crease is where you feel the top of the eyeball.

3. Next, line the upper lashes with a dark, waterproof liner.

4. Finish with waterproof or tube technology (smudge-resisting) mascara on only the top lashes.

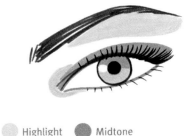

○ Highlight ● Midtone

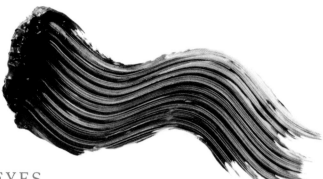

CLOSE-SET EYES

Electrify your intense gaze by using light-toned shadows on the inside half of the lid.

1. First, sweep a highlight shadow across the entire lid, from the lash line to under the brow, making sure to include the inner corners.

2. Next, blend on a midtone eye shadow, starting at the outer half of the lid at the lash line and blending up into the crease.

3. Now, line the eyes starting at the midpoint of the lid and working outward. Repeat on the lower lash line.

4. Follow with mascara, and watch your eyes light up a room.

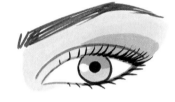

Highlight   Midtone

WIDE-SET EYES

Give your wide, sexy eyes the definition they deserve.

1. Start by applying a highlight shadow only under the brows.

2. Next, take a midtone eye shadow and sweep it across the entire lid, from the lash line and up into the crease.

3. Now, take your eyeliner and start drawing at the inner corners of the eyes, tapering off as you move outward so the line is thickest at the inner corners and thinnest at the outer edges. Blend over this line with an angle brush or a cotton swab for a slightly smudgier look.

4. Follow with mascara, and you're far-out fabulous.

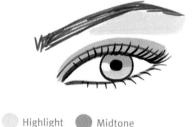

Highlight   Midtone

Mirror Mantra

I absolutely love the sparkle in my green eyes when I'm feeling feisty! They're like emeralds in the sunshine.

Brandy, 43, Santa Rosa, CA

Carmindy Fan Q&A

Q: *I don't know how to play up my brown eyes. I have auburn hair and fair skin but don't like the purple and pink shades that people suggest.*

—Christy, 35, Pomona, CA

A: Try contrasting eyeliner and warm eye shadows for superintense eyes. Start with deep sapphire blue eyeliner smudged across your upper lash line. This deep blue will be a great contrast to your brown eyes and will give them an electrifying jolt. Then, sweep a bronzy copper eye shadow across the lid, and blend some under your lower lash line. Follow with the palest gold highlight under the brow and on the inside corners of the eyes. Finish with black mascara, and watch your eyes ignite!

Q: *I love my Asian eyes. However, my lashes don't seem to hold a curl after using a lash curler and mascara. Any tips?*

—Karen, 29, Great Meadows, NJ

A: Try using a corner eyelash curler instead of the classic full-fringe ones. These sectional curlers offer more control in smaller areas for a stronger effect. Follow immediately with waterproof or tube technology mascara; they keep the curl much longer than regular formulas.

Q: *I love my yellow green-colored eyes; they're unusual and look amazing when I wear purple eye shadow. However, the skin under my eyes sometimes looks thin and crepe paper-like. Is there any way to conceal darkness without accentuating these fine lines?*

—Lisa, 21, San Jose, CA

A: Purples are perfect for playing up those peepers. You can also try emerald green for flirty variety. As for the under-eye crepe paper, I suspect you're trying too hard to conceal a minimal amount of darkness with the maximum amount of concealer. (Chances are nobody notices this darkness but you!) Try gently applying a very thin veil of light pink brightening concealer to make you look awake and refreshed, not masked and crepey.

Q: *I always wear dark blue eyeglasses. Which eye shadows should I use for dark brown eyes while wearing them?*

—Cassie, 22, Evergreen Park, IL

A: I usually say opposites attract when using eye shadows for brown eyes, but since your frames are dark blue, you've got that covered. Try playing with shades of silvery taupe, burgundy, or bronze to make your brown beauties pop.

Q: *As I age, I notice my lids looking heavier. Would using just primer and a highlighter instead of shadows be okay?*

—Rita, 54, Helena, MT

A: You're not alone, sister. The best approach is to embrace your new bedroom eyes and play into them. Keeping shadows to the minimum is the perfect way to go. Try applying an eye shadow base/primer to the lid, then dusting a slight amount of translucent powder on top. Follow with a glowing highlight powder eye shadow under the brow, on the very center of the lid, and on the inside corner of the eyes. Sweep a slight line of waterproof eyeliner on the upper lash line, and follow with a stay-put mascara. Sultry and sexy.

Q: *I love how my eyes sometimes look blue and other times appear gray. What shades should I play with?*

—Tasha, 23, Louisville, KY

A: To boost the blue, choose eye shadows in chocolate browns and burgundies. To go gray, play with silvery taupes and purpleish quartz shades.

Q: *My eyebrows are a little on the unruly side. How can I tame them to best accentuate and frame my long lashes?*

—Jodi, 40, Richland, WA

A: First, brush them up with a brow brush and trim any strays with cuticle scissors. Next, hold your tweezers vertically alongside the bridge of your nose to determine where your brow should start. Pluck any hairs in that unibrow section. Now, hold the tweezers alongside your nose and angle it diagonally so it passes over your iris. This is where the brow should arch; pluck the hairs under this section. Finally, hold the tweezers alongside your nose and angle it outward toward the end of your eye; this is where the brow should end. Clean up above and below this area for a flawless frame.

Q: *I love my big, brown, droopy, puppy-dog eyes. When I talk, they sparkle! I wear glasses and would like to know how to play up my eyes so they shine through. I'm fifty-two and look damn good! Age is only a big number, and just because you act your age, you don't have to look it.*

—Carol, 52, Toronto, ON

A: Way to go, Carol! If you want your lovely eyes to flash through those frames, try applying a luminescent champagne highlighter under the brows and on the inside corners of the eyes. Then, line the upper lash line with waterproof gel eyeliner in sparkling brown, sapphire blue, forest green, or deep plum. Apply one coat of waterproof or tube technology mascara, and glow forth.

Q: *I have deep gray eyes and have never been able to determine the best colors for enhancing them. Any ideas?*

—Betsey, 29, Newport News, VA

A: I suggest lining the eyes with deep amethyst eyeliner and following with a simple sweep of purple shadow across the lid and smudged under the lash line. This will make your gray eyes look mystical and enchanting.

Q: *I love that my eyes are a deep navy, but I need help finding a flattering eye shadow. My complexion is quite pale.*

—Rebecca, 26, Manchester, CT

A: Oooh, that sounds beautiful. Try a sweep of silvery taupe across the lid, and line them with a deep, dark brown. Stupendous!

Q: *I love how my blonde and brunette girlfriends can really play up their eye makeup. I have strawberry blonde hair, green eyes, and fair skin and seem to have trouble mimicking their look without looking overdone.*

—Brittany, 27, Boise, ID

A: First off, stop with the mimicking! Embrace your unique coloring, and let the stunning begin. Play into the warmth of your hair and feature your emerald eyes and pale skin. Try warm eye shadow shades in browns, coppers, bronzes, and golds; line the eyes with chocolate brown or deep purple. Boost your lips and cheeks with peachy shades for a polished look.

Q: *Without looking like Joan Crawford, how can I use a pencil to fill in my short eyebrows?*

—Norma, 41, Seville, Spain

A: Make sure the pencil is very sharp and the shade is right before starting. If you have light hair, choose a brow pencil that matches its darkest strands. If your hair is dark, go one shade lighter than your hair. Use swift feathering motions to fill in the brow and lengthen the ends to where you want them. If you feel like you have overdone it, you can either soften over the top with a cotton swab or use a small-tipped concealer brush to clean up the edges.

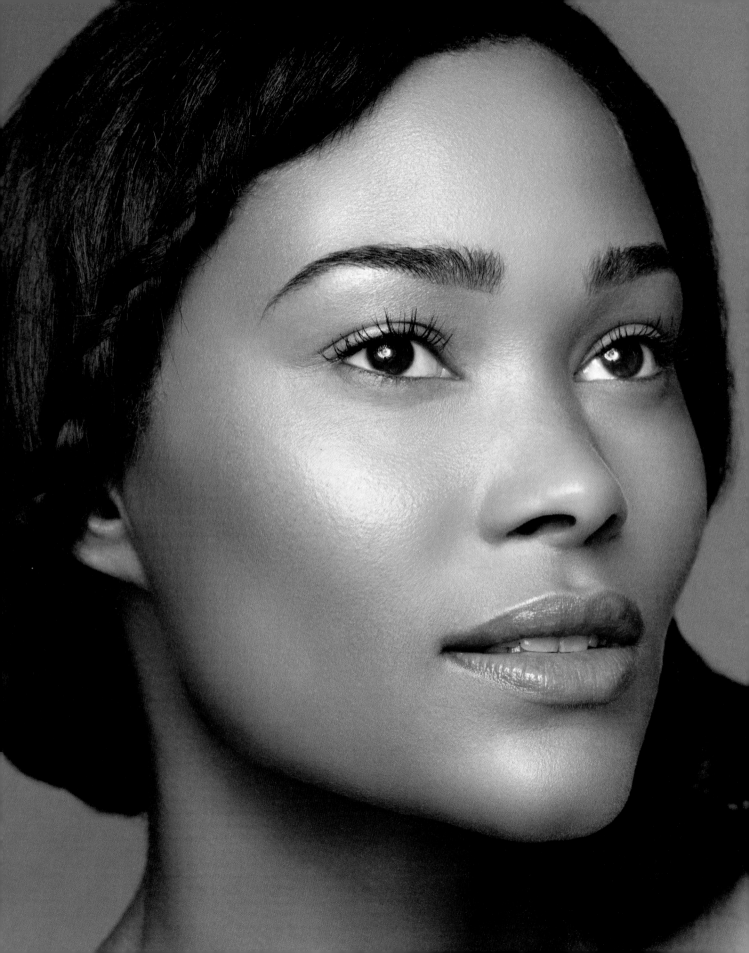

We must be willing to get rid of the life we've planned, so as to have the life that is waiting for us. The old skin has to be shed before the new one can come.

—JOSEPH CAMPBELL

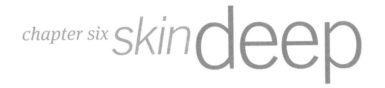

chapter six skin deep

Our skin is more than our shell; it's our storyteller. It gives clues to our heritage, our passions, and our travels in this journey called life. Every laugh line, every scar, every freckle reveals something about who we are and how we've lived. When folks say beauty is only skin deep, we might want to pause and respond. Yes indeed, but skin is also deep; it's wondrous, wonderful, and says so much.

A gorgeously radiant and supple complexion is an outstanding feature to focus on. Whether we're young or advanced in years, we can honor our skin and help it look its best with loving care and the right make-up. From milk-chocolate mahogany to peaches and cream porcelain, every skin tone and type can and should be celebrated.

In my experience, however, skin is a focal point of complaint for most women. I can almost hear you, dear reader, criticizing your own hardworking epidermis. Well, let's get those beefs out in the open so we can bury 'em and move on!

First, pore obsession has become utterly insane and is a poor use of our energies. It's as if women have started removing their bathroom sinks so they can get an inch from the mirror to find these "flawed" little openings in the skin. Companies are all too happy to respond to this madness with hot scrubs, harsh stripping tapes, and other crazy treatments to unblock or shrink pores. Ladies, nobody sees the trouble here but you. Step back

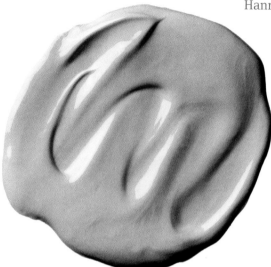

and stop it already! A regular cleansing routine is all your pores want and need. On behalf of pores everywhere, hear their plea: Leave us be!

Second, age-related changes command too much of our time and attention. As adolescents, breakouts break our spirits; as adults, fine lines and unevenness get tracked on an unkind scorecard in a game we should refuse to play. I mean, honestly, if we live, we change. Your skin's texture will evolve with every decade, so how about we try some acceptance and relax? Focus on loving the skin you're in right now, and I guarantee you'll look and feel better.

Embracing your complexion includes finding the right products to showcase its creamy dreaminess. Today's cosmetics are better than ever at boosting luminosity and helping you create a flawless backdrop for the rest of your fantastic features. Playing up your skin and leaving the rest of your makeup simple and natural can be such a sophisticated statement. And what an amazing testament to your confidence!

Here's the skinny on how to make it happen . . .

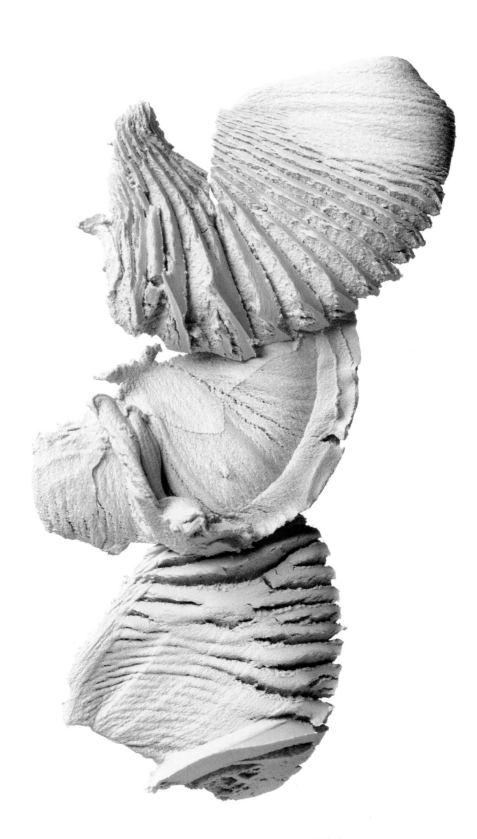

The Goods

PRIMER

Primer is a creamy liquid or gel that is applied as a base layer before foundation. It smoothes out your skin's texture and creates a satiny canvas for foundation to adhere to.

Primer can be beneficial for every skin type. It transforms dry patches into velvety areas, makes oily spots more matte (a lifesaver for oily skin), and helps foundation stay fresh and clean-looking all day. As an added bonus, most primers contain skin-brightening ingredients that enhance your radiance and complement the look and feel of your foundation.

FOUNDATION

Foundation is *the* go-to product to achieve the ultimate in polished, perfected skin. It's also often the toughest challenge in the makeup aisle. So many choices! Small differences in shade and/or texture can make a world of difference in your overall look.

To find the right foundation for you, first test the color by applying a stripe of it onto your jawline, not the back of your hand. Then have a look in natural light. Did it blend well with your complexion's tone? Does it feel good on your skin? If so, go for it.

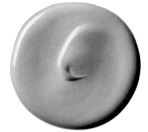

Liquid foundation — These are my favorite because they just melt onto the skin and blend beautifully. The right liquid foundation mimics your skin's natural texture while smoothing out any unevenness, boosting your overall appearance.

Tinted moisturizer — A good choice for women who want the faintest hint of coverage plus a hydrating supplement for suppleness. Most tinted moisturizers also contain sunscreen, making them a triple threat of benefits.

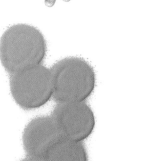

Spray foundation — Ideal for women who need a bit heavier and longer-wearing coverage.

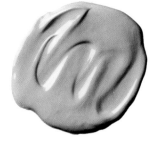

Cream foundation — Best for women with very dry skin; this formulation is a bit too heavy for other skin types.

No matter which foundation you choose, the key word for pristine results is *blend*. Say it loud, and make it so. Heck, make a cheer out of it: B-L-E-N-D, *Be Lovely Every New Day, Okay!* Blend on your foundation lightly and lovingly; we want to see your skin, not a mask.

CONCEALER

Hmmm . . . concealer. Even the word is suspect. We're not here to hide a darn thing about your beauty. Maybe we should rename it "focus shifter" instead. Concealer is often abused; let's rethink it and go easy.

Two types of concealer *can* help spotlight your awesome complexion: under-eye concealer and blemish concealer.

Under-eye concealer — This should have a pinky or peachy undertone and should be bright and lightly applied. Use it to illuminate the under-eye area, giving your eyes that fresh, wide-awake look. If you try to erase every last trace of darkness, you'll wind up with a creasy, cakey mess.

Blemish concealer — This has recently appeared in crazy colors like purple and green. Now, unless you're Michelangelo, good luck trying to blend them into the right combination. For concealing minor imperfections, choose a concealer that is about a half shade lighter than your foundation and has a more yellow cast instead of a pinky undertone. Pat it on lightly, and remember that you're a supercharged lady who won't let a little zit zap your style.

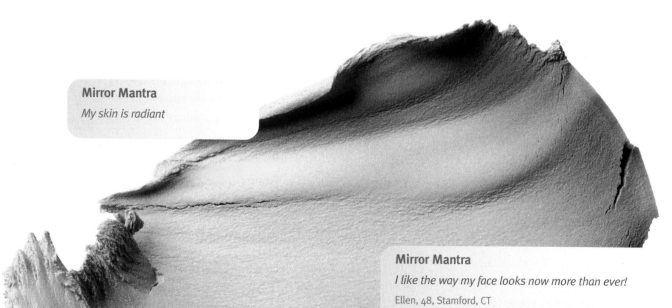

Mirror Mantra

My skin is radiant

Mirror Mantra

I like the way my face looks now more than ever!
Ellen, 48, Stamford, CT

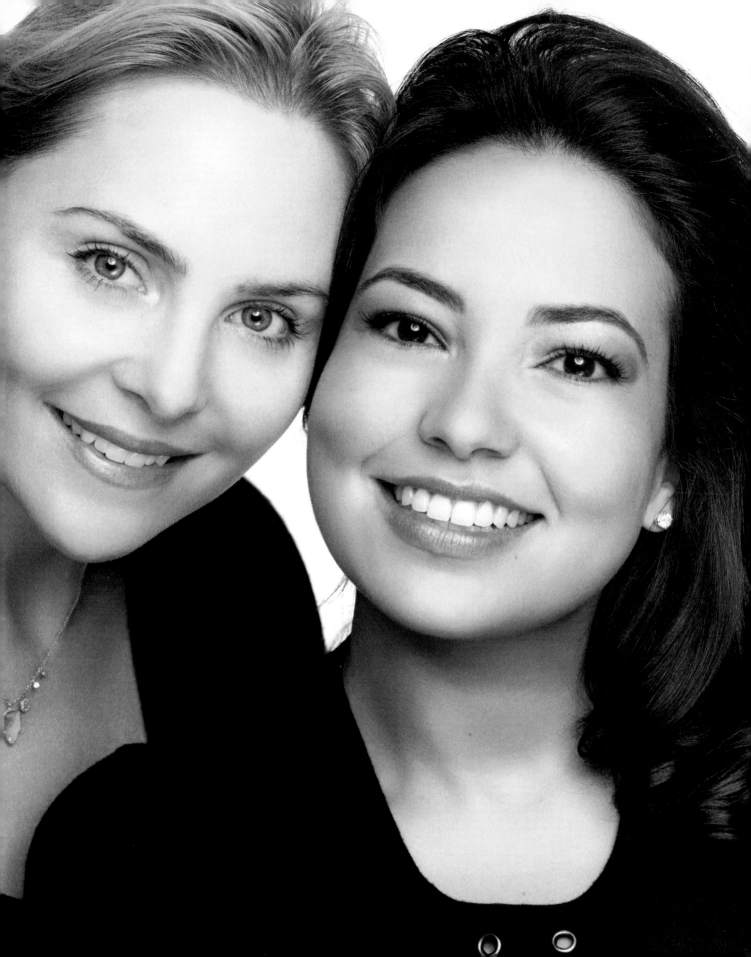

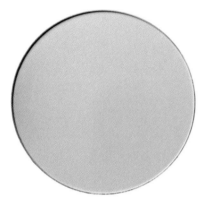

POWDER

Powder eliminates shine and sets your makeup so it will last all day. Texture is everything; you don't want to add a heavy layer to your smooth skin. Always choose a sheer, finely milled powder. Stay away from skin-brightening sparkle formulas; they're overpowering and can age older skin. Leave the brightening work to highlighter.

I like to apply loose powder with a puff or pressed powder with a powder brush for precise placement and a sheer finish.

HIGHLIGHTER

Highlighter draws attention to the skin with a touch of light-catching shimmer. As we discussed in the last chapter and will touch on more in the next, highlighter is key to the "Carmindy look" and creates a taut-looking, amazing glow. Whether cream or powder, a dab of highlighter on the cheekbones or temples or brow bone—wherever you want to captivate—is simply sizzling!

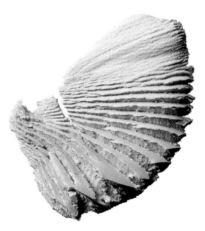

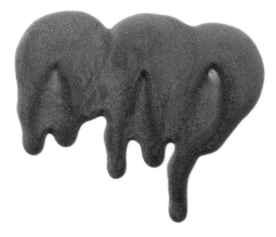

BRONZER

Fake the bake! Bronzer is the only way to go when you want a sun-kissed look. Take your time and blend, blend, blend so you look marvelous, not muddy. Go for creams for a natural, subtle look; powders for more of a kick; and sprays for an all-over bronze that remains gloriously golden for hours and hours.

Put a Fresh Face on Your Look

Most women have a set makeup routine for their skin and only have fun modifying their look by playing up eyes, lips, and/or cheeks. However, your complexion can be the focal point for an entirely fresh appearance. If you're in the mood to say buh-bye to boring, give these surefire techniques a try.

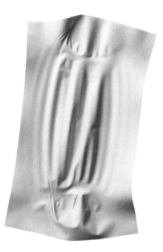

DEWY SKIN

Think fresh, natural, and youthful. Dewy is, in a word, divine!

The trick here is after you apply your primer, foundation, and concealer, skip face powder in a few key places. Leave the top of the cheekbones, center of the forehead, bridge of the nose, and chin free of powder. Your skin's natural oils will give your face a glow all its own.

If you have very oily skin, use blotting papers throughout the day to zip away any excess oil. If your skin is extra dry, try dabbing on the tiniest bit of cream highlighter just on the top of the cheekbones.

SATINY MATTE SKIN

Some women still love the retro chic, matte look. But let's take a more modern approach. The key is in the placement of satiny sheer, finely milled powder. This will give you a refined, elegant appearance without any of that old-school chalkiness.

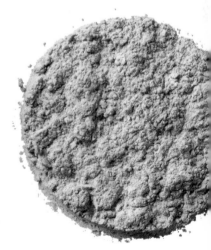

After your applying primer, foundation, and concealer, dust loose powder lightly over your entire face for a satiny finish. Skip the highlighter. If you want a subtle bronze sheen, sweep on shimmerless bronzer.

If your skin becomes a bit oily throughout the day, use blotting papers first to soak up any shine; if necessary, lightly apply some pressed powder for a velvety soft finish.

SUN-KISSED BRONZED SKIN

Oh goodness, oh goddess!

Start with primer, foundation, concealer, and powder to set the stage for golden gloriousness. Next, apply powder bronzer on the sides of the forehead, along the temples, and under the cheekbones. This frames the planes of your face. You can blend a slight amount onto the center of the forehead and across the bridge of your nose, but take extra care to blend it well.

I never apply bronzer over the entire face or on the chin; it tends to look a bit dirty, so be strategic! Keep your cheeks free for blush that will later complement the bronzer.

If you use spray or cream bronzers, apply them before face powder to keep the skin looking clean, fresh, and natural. For spray bronzer, first spritz it onto a nonlatex sponge, then apply; for cream bronzer, use a nonlatex sponge, your fingers, or a bronzer brush.

Bronzers vary in their level of sparkle. Younger women can choose bronzers with a bit of shimmer, and mature gals should stick with nonsparkling formulas.

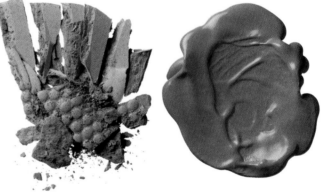

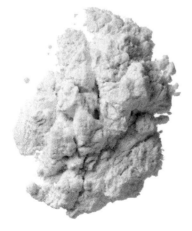

SHIMMER AND GLOW SKIN

Festive, ethereal, and so unbelievably alluring!

Highlighter is the crucial product for this look. First, apply your primer, foundation, concealer, and powder. Then, starting at the temples, sweep shimmering highlighter down and across the top of your cheekbones in a C formation. (If you use cream highlighter, apply it before the powder.)

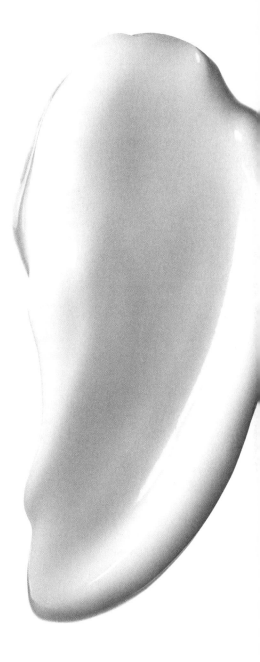

For extra drama, you can add a bit of highlighter to the center of the forehead, along the bridge of the nose, and on the chin. This brings a galaxy of light to your face, so your skin is the star. (When choosing highlighter, remember that mature skin looks best with a cream formula that does not contain shimmer.)

For a fast, subtle, all-over glow, just mix a bit of liquid shimmer into your foundation for a soft sheen.

BODY BARING MAGIC

Whether you're showing off your treasure chest of décolletage, wearing a shoulder-baring top, or working a leggy mini, your body's skin deserves enhancing treats, too!

After showering, apply moisturizer to your entire hot bod, then smooth or spray on a bit of body shimmer. Sprays go on fast and easy—no need to rub them in—and usually dry quickly. With creams, blend all over or focus on your favorite, attention-grabbing areas. Powdered shimmers are fine, too, but make sure your moisturizer is fully absorbed first. Avoid any bronze-tinted shades if you're donning light-colored clothing.

The magically glowing result will not only leave you looking radiant, your skin will instantly appear more taut and toned. How's that for an awesome workout?

Mirror Mantra

I tell myself, "Anne, you were beautiful at twenty, incredible at thirty, and forty is just amazing!" I embrace whatever age skin I'm in!
Anne, 40, Methuen, MA

Savor Skin Care as a Beauty Ritual

What's particularly thrilling about skin is how responsive it is to attention. Think of it as similar to a child—constantly changing and developing in lockstep with great nurturing, proper nutrition, and motherly protection. Your skin loves to be loved!

Embrace your skin care regimen as a time to care for your tender wrappings. We all know the steps, but they bear repeating because they work wonders when practiced religiously. Remember, you don't have to pay outrageous prices for effective skin care products. Today's drugstore brands feature many of the same active ingredients as boutique potions. What matters is making skin care a daily ritual you enjoy.

The tried-and-true basics:

- Cleanse with a gentle facial cleanser each morning, follow with a moisturizer suitable for your skin type, and add a topper of sunscreen. Many moisturizers now come with an SPF conveniently built right in. (Winter or summer, sunny or cloudy, sunscreen is *mandatory.*)

- Cleanse again at night, removing any stubborn makeup with makeup remover, and apply a replenishing night cream before bed. If you experience breakouts, bedtime is the right time to apply a drying solution to blemishes—gently, and no picking, please. Eye cream is another luxurious little treat to tap on before your beauty sleep. Finish with a slick of lip balm to maintain your dreamy pucker.

- Exfoliating your skin is the best way to keep it soft and evenly textured. I recommend exfoliating a couple of times a week with a mixture of your daily cleanser and white sugar to rid your face of dead skin cells, dry patches, and built-up sebum. Your skin will be smooth as glass, and makeup will blend easier.

• For a healthy glow, you have to nourish your insides as well. Eat a lot of fresh fruits, vegetables, and foods containing Omega-3 oils like salmon. Pop a multivitamin or anti-oxidant supplement every day for extra insurance. Breathe deeply to relieve stress and calm your spirit. Drink plenty of water and choose green tea over coffee or sodas. Make sure to exercise regularly to get the blood pumping. This helps remove impurities and aids in cell renewal.

• Most important, praise your skin for doing such a fantastic job. It literally keeps us together, ladies. That's the kind of skin-deep beauty to appreciate!

Mirror Mantra
If I take care of my skin, it will continue to take care of me!
Tara, 30, Upper Marlboro, MD

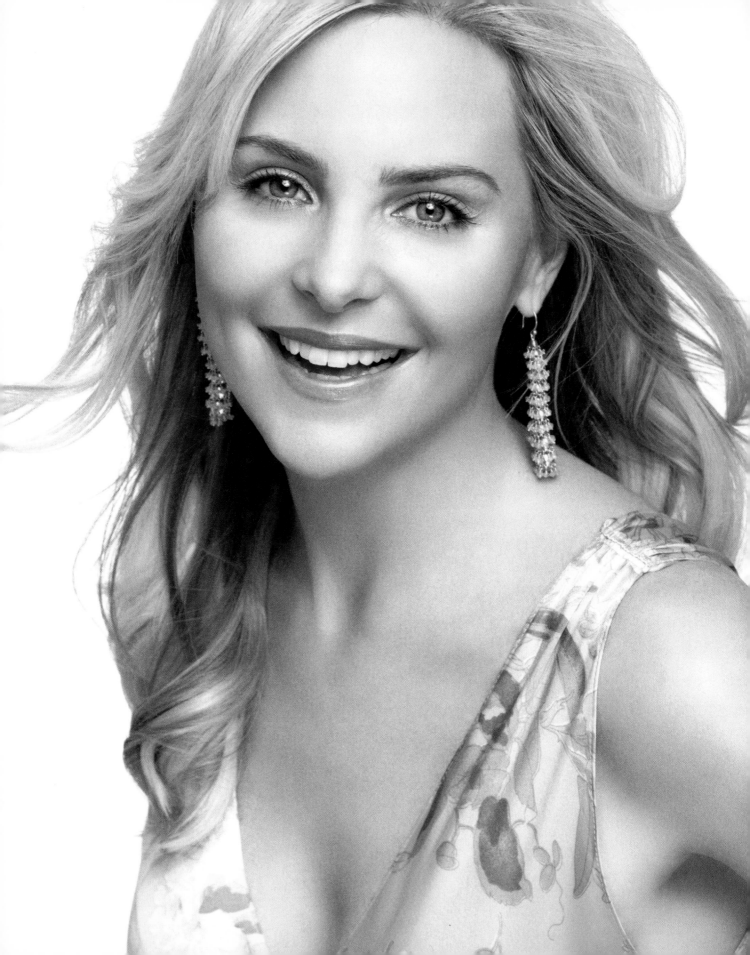

Carmindy Fan Q&A

Q: *How can I make my aging skin look smooth and even-toned without looking heavily made up?*

—Becky, 49, Peotone, IL

A: The trick here is to choose the right foundation. Go for a liquid formula that melts right into your skin for a natural finish. Stay away from heavy concealers and powders that dull the skin. Using a skin-brightening primer before applying foundation is another great way to ensure a smooth and youthful appearance.

Q: *Being in my late twenties, I'm eager to find a skin-care solution that provides sun protection plus ingredients that combat wrinkles (thinking ahead).*

—Theresa, 28, Toronto, ON

A: Sunscreen is your first line of defense against those damaging, aging rays. Choose a moisturizer with a built-in sunscreen to protect yourself in one easy step. Look for makeup containing antioxidants (great age fighters) and other natural skin care goodies like papaya and cork oak extracts that nourish your skin and help keep it in tip-top shape.

Q: *How can I make my skin glow without looking too oily?*

—Hayley, 23, Sammamish, WA

A: Apply a powder highlight only in key areas, not all over your face. Sweep it on top of the cheekbones, under the brows, and on the inside corners of the eyes. Your skin will glow without looking greasy.

Q: *How do I best cover both blemishes and tiny acne scars?*

—Monica, 25, Tama, IA

A: A light touch is key; applying too much concealer draws attention. I suggest using a small-tipped concealer brush to dab on a little blemish concealer mixed with a bit of your regular foundation. Use the fine tip of the brush to apply a bit of this mixture, then lightly blend the edges with the brush. Take a cotton swab dipped in a little translucent powder and dab the area to set it.

Q: *As an African American, I love my caramel complexion and would love to play it up with not just warm colors, but cool ones as well. Should I?*

—Danielle, 35, Philadelphia, PA

A: With your beautiful skin tone, you have a lot more color choices than most women. When choosing cool shades, go deep or bold, but skip pastels—they can look ashy against your complexion. Think in terms of jewel tones, like amethyst, emerald, and navy blue for eyes; for cheeks and lips, try bold pinks, berries, or deep plums.

Q: *How can I cancel the red tint in my older eyelids?*

—Darla, 56, Boise, ID

A: That's an easy one. Just tap a little eye shadow base onto the lid. It neutralizes the red and helps shadows stay truer longer.

Q: *I'm a former sun worshipper and am now paying the price with dark patches around my jawline. Foundation doesn't cover them, and I've tried several skin lighteners without success. Suggestions?*

—Cindy, 47, Tallahassee, FL

A: This is a call for your dermatologist. There are wonderful new procedures to reverse serious sun damage, such as glycolic peels and lasers. But only a professional dermo should perform them. After treatment, you must be extra diligent about applying sunscreen, or the dark patches will return. In the meantime, stop trying to mask the area with heavy foundation. Instead, brighten your whole complexion by applying a light-reflecting primer before foundation.

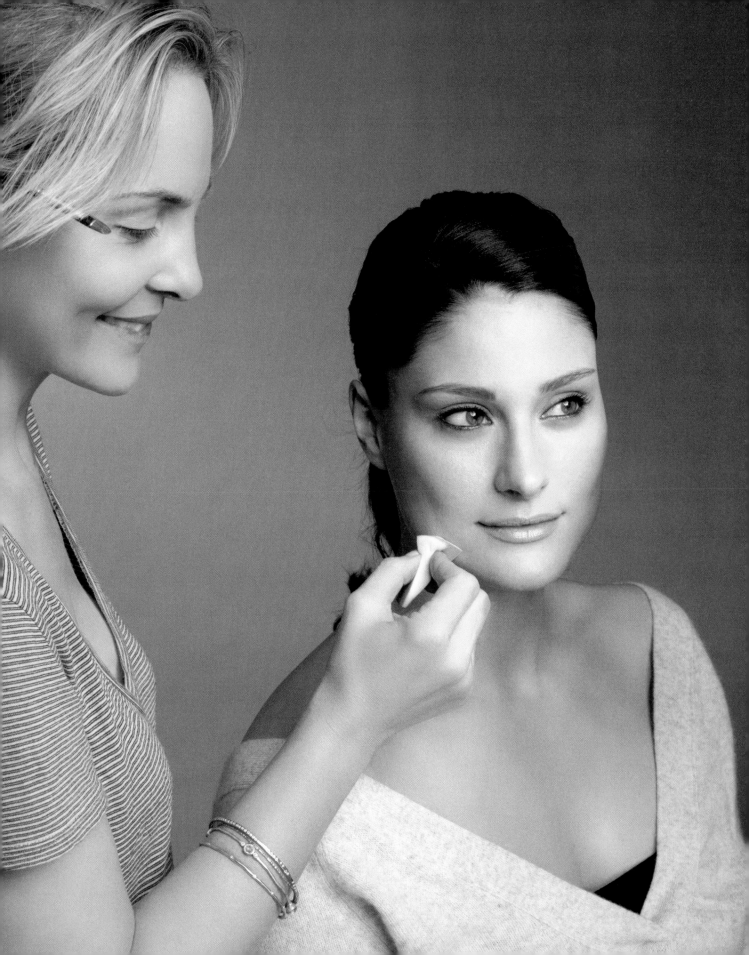

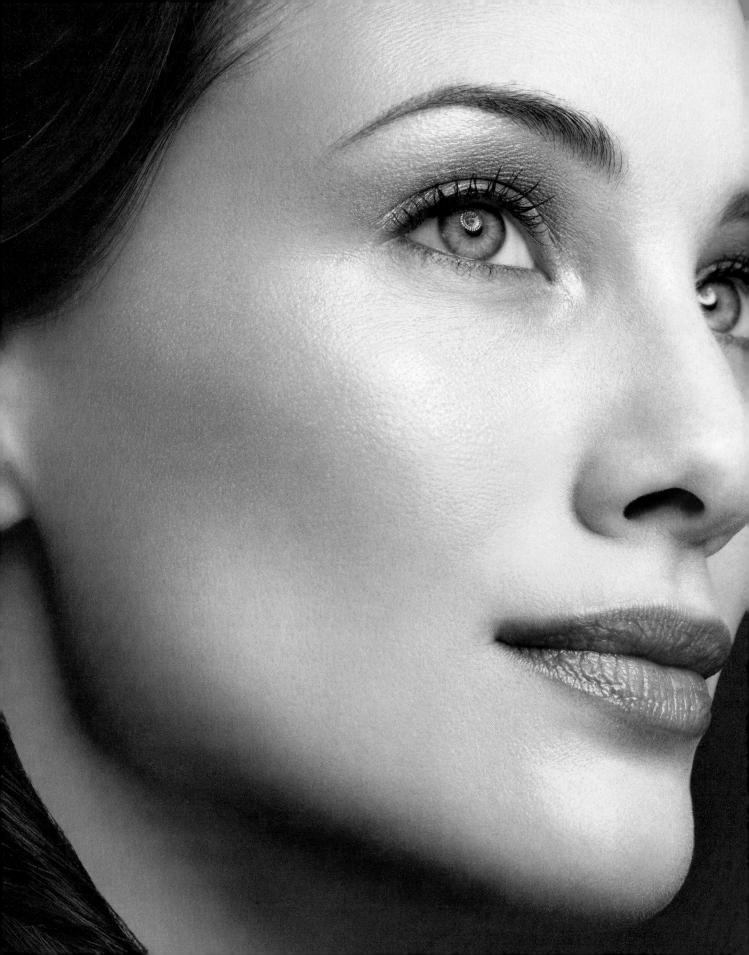

Truth is beauty, beauty truth.

—JOHN KEATS

chapter seven getting cheeky

Great cheeks are absolutely adorable. When we're feeling healthy and strong, they bloom with vitality. When we're swept up in a new love, they get all rosy with bliss. When we're lost in laughter, their dimples and roundness sing out our happiness. Cheeks often play second fiddle to other features, but with so much zing to offer, we should reconsider cheeks as potential stars for a fresh, new look.

With the right touch of makeup, your cheeks can serve as an expressive canvas. Play up the apples to boost the natural glow of your grin. Or focus on the angular shadows of your cheekbones to deepen your vixen allure. Whether round or flat, high or low, your cheeks expand with your smile, bring balance to your face and— look out—encourage kisses!

If cheeks are your feature focus, enjoy enhancing them with new techniques or an expanded product palette. When choosing the best formulas, consider that normal skin accepts most anything, dry skin should head for creams, oily skin fares best with powders and sprays, and smooth, even skin plays well with gels.

Just remember: go easy with the rest of your makeup so you shine, not blind.

Now let's start getting cheeky!

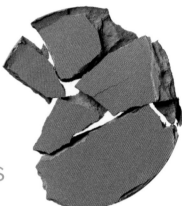

The Goods
BLUSH

Did you know that humans are the only animals that blush? Mark Twain once said that was because we're the only creatures that need to! Well, I say a beautiful flush of natural radiance is far from embarrassing. It's glorious and easily enhanced with today's blushes.

The Colors

Blush brings color to the cheeks, mimics youthful vitality, and can take years off your face. Your complexion is your guide to finding the best blush shade. Fair-skinned beauties should think peach and pink, lovelies with medium-tone skin should go for corals and roses, and for darker-skinned goddesses, the brighter the better in any bold shade or hue.

The Right Type

There are a bevy of blush formula choices—powders, creams, stains, and gels—so if you haven't tried something new in a while, now's the time to experiment. As for finishes, sheer matte or sparkling shimmer? Perhaps both—one for daytime demure, one for nighttime glamour. One general rule is to stick with matte formulas if you're over forty or have facial scars. This keeps the focus on the vivifying color.

The Tools

Achieve blush application perfection with the right tools. For powder blush, use a large powder brush with natural hairs. This size brush hugs the cheeks and whisks the color on for a flawless finish. Creams, stains, and gels are best applied with your fingertips in small, circular motions; always apply them after foundation but before powder.

For more details on brushes and tools, see chapter ten, Tool Time.

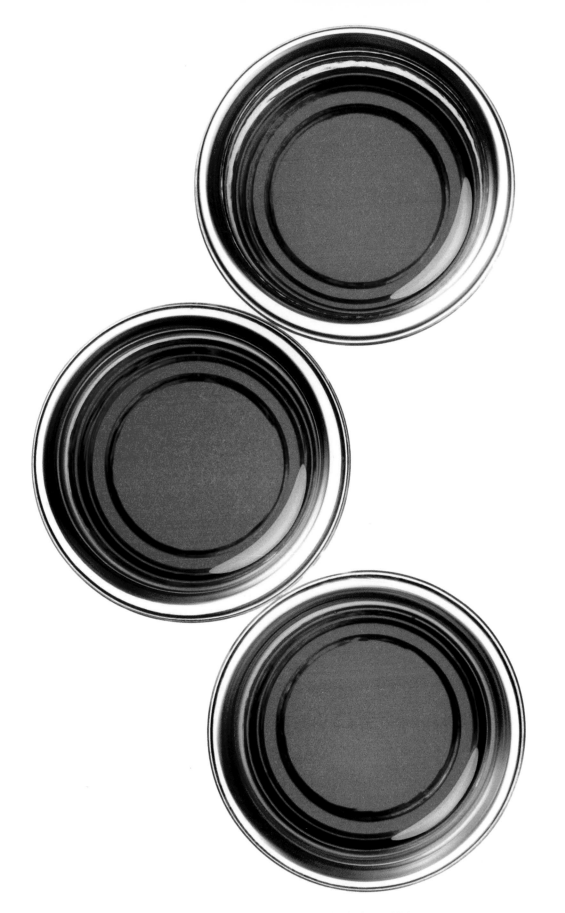

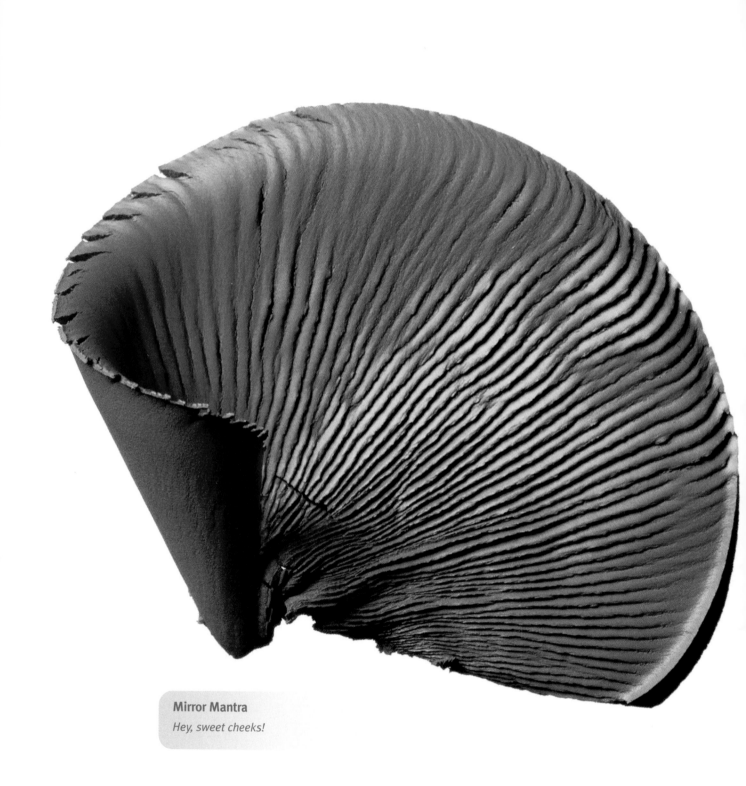

Mirror Mantra

Hey, sweet cheeks!

HIGHLIGHTER

The miracle of highlighter, discussed in the chapter on eyes, can also work wonders for your cheeks. Highlighter draws attention to the tops of your cheekbones, enhancing their form while creating a shimmering luminosity. That little hint of light will attract the gaze of all who take in your amazing cheekbones. Outstanding!

Highlighters come in powders and creams and are best used sparingly. A highlighting eye shadow can just as easily be used for the tops of the cheekbones. My favorite way to apply highlighter is to lightly dot on cream formulas with the fingers or swirl on powdered highlighters with a fan brush. If you have mature skin or an uneven complexion, use a bit of cream all-over brightener without shimmer to achieve a brilliant result.

BRONZER

Bronzers are an excellent replacement for blush when you want a natural, sun-kissed look. If you're in the mood for high drama, bring on a triple play of bronzer, blush, and highlighter to really take your cheeks to the next level.

Bronzers come in creams, powders, and sprays and look best when applied with a light hand and *lots of blending.* (Can we agree that stripes aren't sexy?) I like to use a wide-angle, natural-hair brush to apply powders, a wide-angle, synthetic-hair brush for creams, and a nonlatex sponge for sprays. A little bronzer goes a long way toward tropical tremendous!

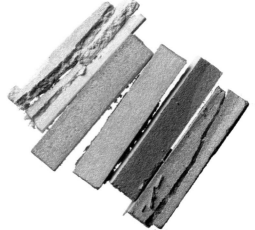

If you go a little overboard on blush, there's no need to start over. Tone cream blush by dipping a sponge in a bit of foundation and buffing the cheeks gently to blend. For powder blush, use a powder brush that has been dipped into a bit of loose powder to turn the color down a notch.

Techniques for Charming Cheeks

Many women express distress with their cheeks, claiming they are too chubby or too sunken or simply unremarkable. Could we please put that negative tape on permanent pause? Or, even better, could we instead revel in these two expressive spans of skin and bone that support our eyes and widen our smiles?

If you feel a self-critical comment coming on, take a breath and give your pair a kind little pinch. Say, "Oh sweet cheeks, where would I be without you?" Seriously! Your fabulous face is incomplete without the charms of those cheeks.

The following techniques will help you celebrate your cheeks as they are rather than attempt to artificially contour or camouflage them. Try these tricks out, and then go forth and glow, baby!

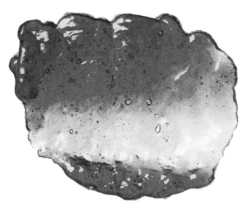

Mirror Mantra

Relax! It keeps you younger on your face and in your soul!

Madeline, 27, San Clemente, CA

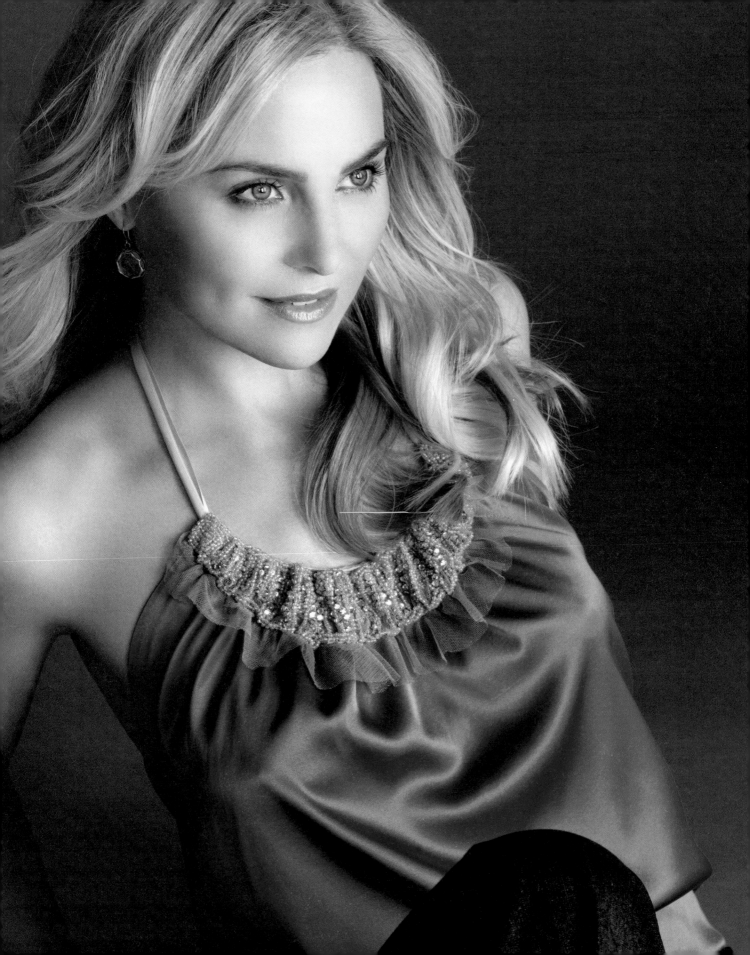

ROUND CHEEKS

Round cheeks are so sweetly cherublike, it pains me when they go underappreciated. When played up in rosy hues and enhanced with a beaming smile, round cheeks are absolutely enchanting.

Start by smiling big and applying blush to the apples (the fleshy part of the cheek) in a swirl of color. Next, add a little highlighter to the outer top of the cheekbones. To find the perfect placement, simply lay your pointer and center fingers side-by-side horizontally under the eye at the outer corner. Under this spot is where you dab on a bit of highlighter. Captivating!

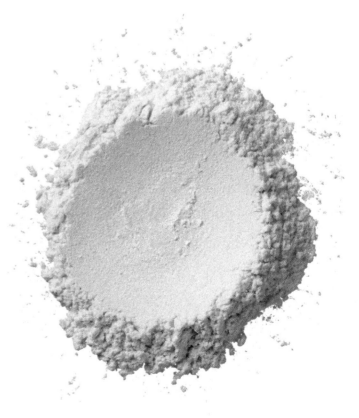

Mirror Mantra

I cannot control how others perceive me; I can only control how I see myself.

Ive, 41, Rego Park, NY

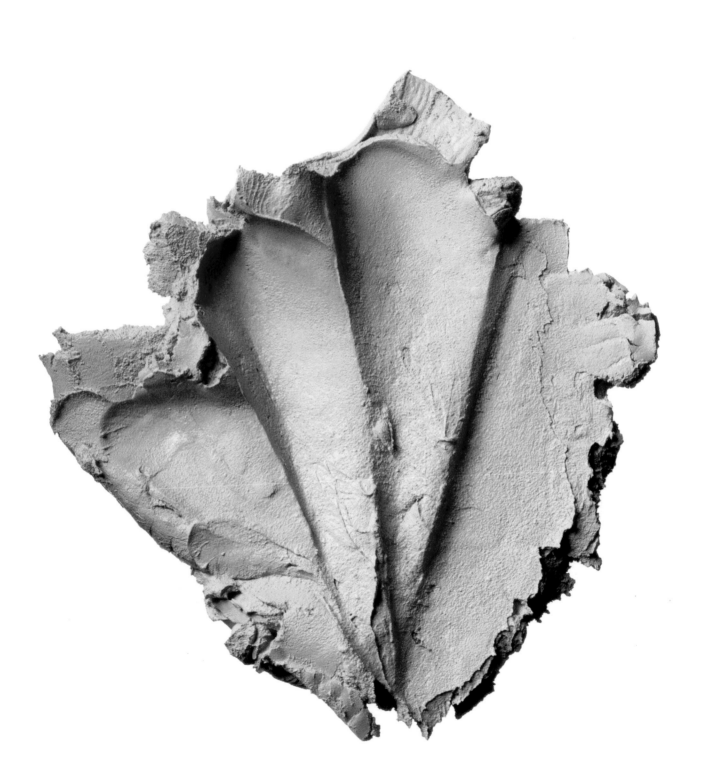

FLAT CHEEKS

Flat cheeks set the scene for a refined, balanced look. A simple three-part technique will define and elevate your elegant cheeks.

First, sweep on highlighter starting along the temples and across the top of the cheekbones, forming a shape like a big letter C. To find the correct area above the cheekbones, put your pointer and center fingers together, and lay them horizontally under the eye at the outer corners. Under this spot is where the highlighter goes to light up the cheekbones and increase their prominence.

Next, sweep blush from the hairline (under the highlighter) toward the nose, stopping two finger-widths away from the nostril.

Finally, suck in your cheeks and lightly sweep a bit of bronzer under the hollows. Start from the side of your face, next to your ears, and brush down and inward. Irresistible!

Mirror Mantra

As a war survivor from Cambodia, I am thankful each day for my life and health. Many others were not so lucky.

Sori, 35, Las Vegas, NV

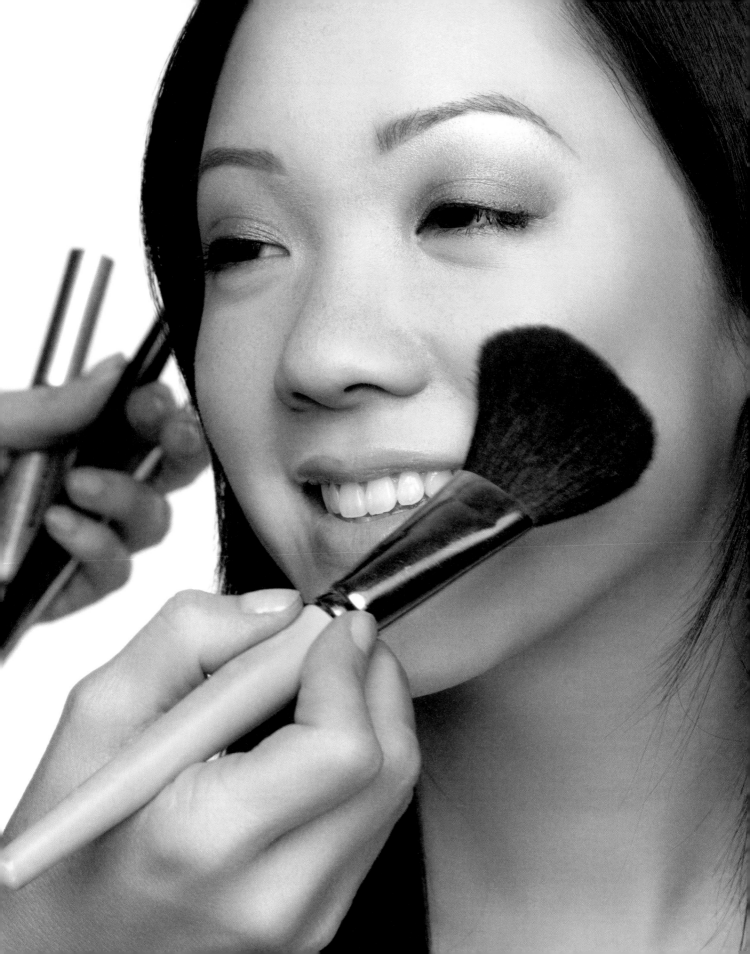

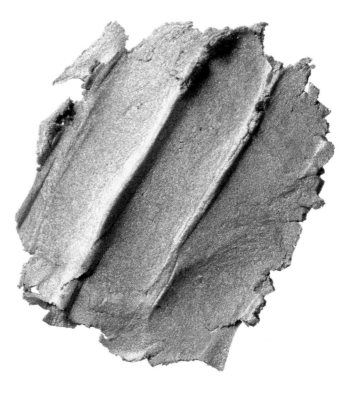

HIGH CHEEKBONES

Intriguing high cheekbones deserve an intensity supercharge. Start by using highlighter along the top of the cheekbones, starting at the temples and sweeping down toward the nose, stopping just three finger-widths away from the nose.

Next, apply blush on the apples of the cheeks, and lightly buff the color outward toward the hairline. Choosing a shimmering blush formula will really showcase these beauties for the ultimate in electrifying ka-pow!

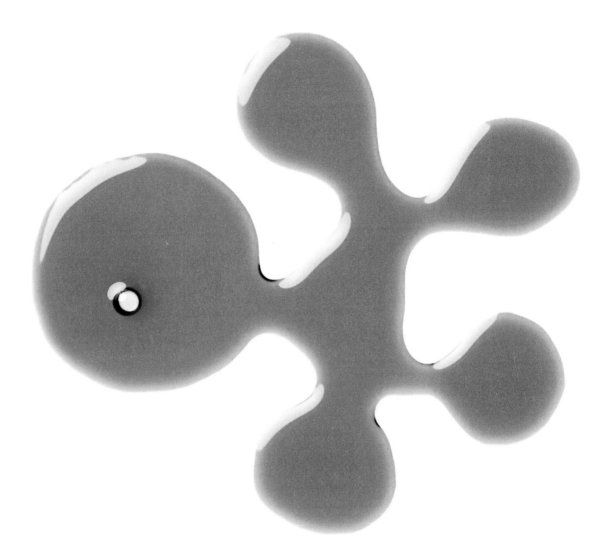

LOW CHEEKBONES

Sultry, low cheekbones can command the limelight. It's as easy as letting your fingers be your guide.

First, apply bright blush two vertical finger-widths away from the nose and two horizontal finger-widths below the eyes. This pop of color brings attention to the cheeks by enhancing the apples.

Next, sweep a bit of highlighter along the temples and on top of the cheekbones at the outer edges. Devastating!

> I love my cheeks. Why? My husband loves to kiss them. He talks about them constantly. It makes me feel beautiful.
> Candice, 27, Collinsville, IL

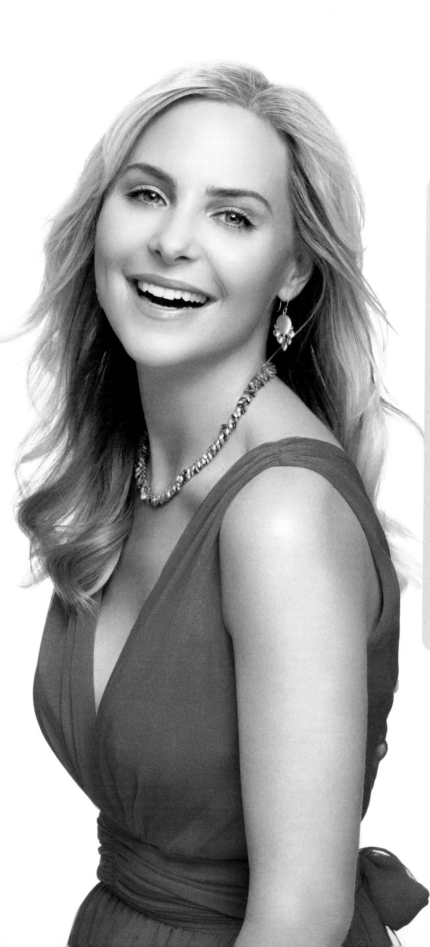

Working with Rosacea

Women with rosacea may choose to forgo blush because they already possess the natural flush the rest of us are trying to evoke. Instead of cursing rosacea, consider it a time-saver in the morning. However, if your rosacea causes the slightest anguish, simply apply foundation and then blend on a little yellow-toned neutralizing concealer over the affected cheek area. This will counteract any extra redness, evening out your skin tone. Dust on a little loose powder, and then choose a light taupe rose shade of blush, and apply in one easy swipe from the apples to the hairline. Lovely!

Carmindy Fan Q&A

Q: *I really like using blush to add more color to my face, but sometimes the redness around my nose area becomes the focus instead of my highlighted cheeks. How can I prevent this?*

—Megan, 23, Glendora, CA

A: By first creating an even skin canvas, your cheeks can command the spotlight. Start with the right foundation, then dab on a red-neutralizing concealer around the nose area. Dust with a little powder, and then swirl on your blush to the cheekbones, but stay at least two finger-widths away from the nose. You'll look energized and polished.

Q: *My cheeks get red in cold weather, making blush look overpowering, yet I need some color when I'm inside. Any ideas?*

—Marian, 63, Brooklyn, NY

A: Lucky you to have a built-in blush! For a more consistent pink in your cheeks, first even out your complexion with a liquid foundation. Next, try a soft shade of cream blush that is a little lighter than your wintertime red flush. Lightly dust powder on top for a soft finish. You'll maintain a subtle indoor blush and won't look like Santa when you're out in the snow.

Q: *I have a round face and would love to show more definition in my cheekbones. I like a paler look, and most bronzers make me look like I'm trying too hard. Maybe a darker blush?*

—Lana, 23, San Francisco, CA

A: Oh, my cheeky darling, it's not the shade but where you place it that makes all the difference. First, spotlight those round cheeks by placing highlighter on top of the cheekbones, sweeping in from the temples and stopping about two finger-widths away from your nose. Next, smile big and swirl rosy blush onto the apples. Now for definition, suck in your cheeks and sweep a softer shade of powder bronzer into the hollows. Lovely!

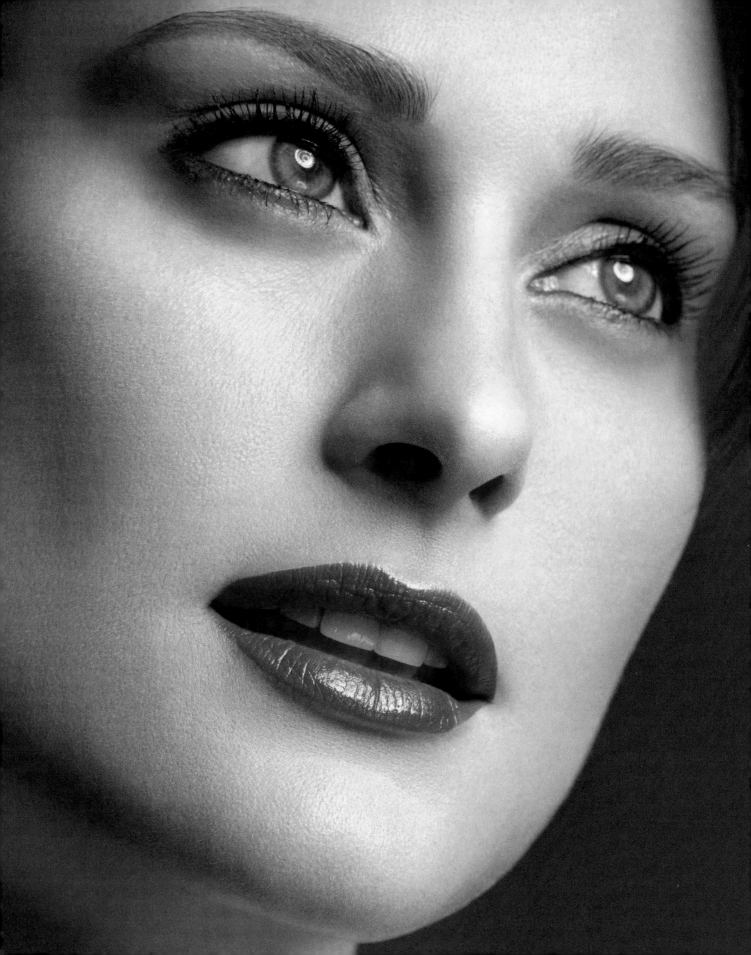

Sometimes your joy is the source of your smile, but sometimes
your smile can be the source of your joy.
—THICH NHAT HANH

chapter eight luscious lips

Lips bring such bliss to our days. Laughter! Tasting a scrumptious dish! Offering an encouraging word! And my personal favorite, kissing! Clearly, our powerhouse puckers deserve pampering.

Too many of us, however, have been caught up in obsessing over changing our lips instead of treating them like treasures. We waste our energy drawing on someone else's idea of the perfect pout or fixate on making lips look bigger to the point of undergoing injections or pouring on burning lip plumpers. Ladies, inflamed, unnaturally large lips appear painful, not pretty, so *enough already*.

Whether small, large, thin, thick, bow-shaped, crooked, or asymmetrical, all lips are beautiful communication billboards. They say so much about each woman's unique character, quirkiness and, yes, sex appeal. Start celebrating your own perfect pair by playing 'em up!

There's something supremely feminine about painting lips with a slick of eye-catching color. If getting luscious lips is your feature focus, get ready to have fun going Picasso! Cosmetics aisles today overflow with great new lip products to enhance your look and light up your smile in seconds. Now *that's* what I call lip service!

The Goods
LIP LINER

Colored lip liners should come with a warning label: Caution, potential for abuse! For years, women have used liners to draw on lips they don't have, to "correct" unevenness that would otherwise look really cute, to attempt to lock in lipstick for twenty-four hours or more, or to seal in gloss only to get "ring around the mouth" in a few hours. Ay-yay-yay.

Now, lip liners do have their place in a lady's lippy repertoire, but easy does it, okay?

To make your lips look their fullest, try one of the new shimmering highlight lip liners. They offer a light-catching hint of sparkle without any distracting color. When traced around the outside of your *natural* lip line, these liners bring out your beauties' plumpest potential.

If you have issues with lipstick bleeding, try a clear or skin-tone lip liner to keep your color from running off in all directions.

Attention, endurance enthusiasts who absolutely hate to reapply lipstick: please be careful of long-wearing formulas. Some of these superstick compounds can dry out your lips, causing chapping and parching. Make sure to choose moisture-rich formulas or try this trick instead. Using a flesh-colored lip liner, trace your natural lip line—softening the edge with a cotton swab—and then fill in the lips with more liner. Finish with a swipe of lipstick for a natural look with staying power.

When I smile, it accentuates my high cheekbones. My husband says that my smile was the first feature he noticed from across the room.
Stephanie, 30, Webster, MA

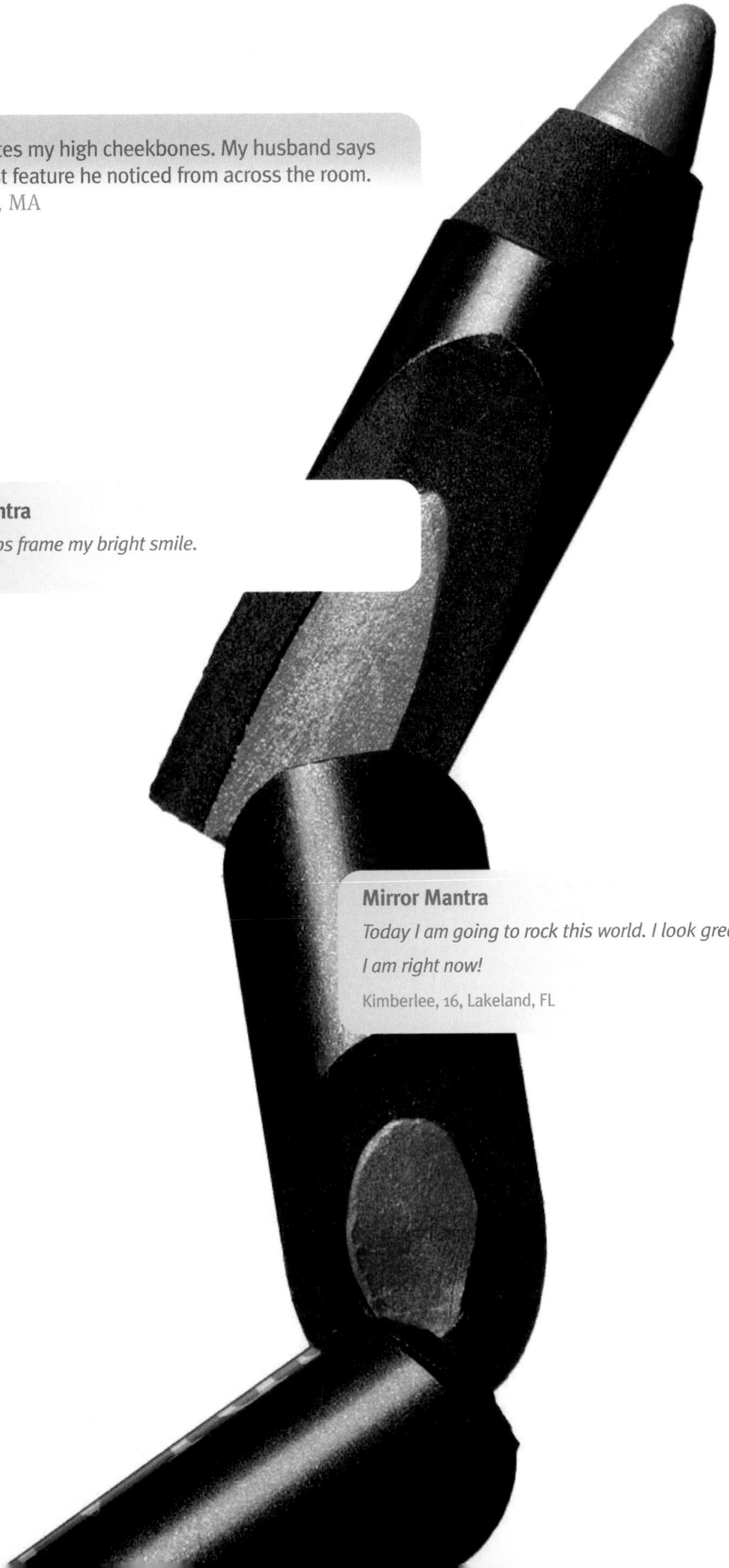

Mirror Mantra

My lovely lips frame my bright smile.

Mirror Mantra

Today I am going to rock this world. I look great as I am right now!

Kimberlee, 16, Lakeland, FL

Bamboozled by color choices? Start with rose lipstick; it complements every skin tone. Redheads look great in warm rose, fair ladies shine in cool pink rose, medium/olive complexions win with true rose, and darker complexions beam with deeper rose.

Banish lipstick traces from your teeth forever. After application, stick your pointer finger into your mouth and close it. Slide your finger out, and off comes the excess that would otherwise wind up on your teeth.

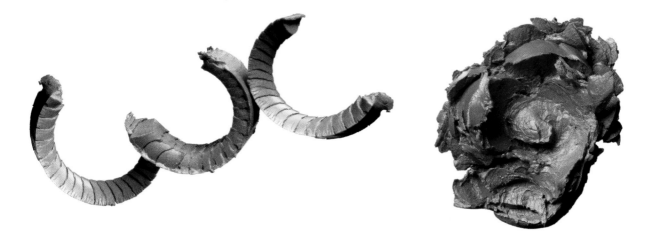

LIPSTICK

Remember playing dress-up and digging in mom's makeup drawer? Chances are your little hands first grabbed for those shiny tubes of big-girl crayons in pretty pinks, reds, and corals. I say let's keep that spirit of play in play. Lipstick remains a great way to dress up the face with a simple flick of the wrist.

Lipstick has recently made a comeback, with a host of rich and moisturizing new formulas that are free from old-school heaviness. Matte, shimmer, pearl, satin—there is definitely a texture and finish out there for you. And, my goodness, what a rainbow of hues. Step out of your color rut, ladies! Today's sheer lipsticks are wonderfully translucent and an ideal choice for experimenting with trendy new shades.

Whether you apply straight from the tube, use a lip brush for precision, or tap the color on your finger, lipstick will showcase your smile like nothing else. There are even lip colors now that make your teeth look whiter and brighter with one easy swipe. Look for lipsticks featuring color pigments that contain blue undertones to make your teeth look their pearly best.

Nutrients, antioxidants, and other yummy skin treats are also showing up in new lipstick formulas. It's about time we focus on the health of our lips and not their size. Hey, while we're at it, let's think that way about *every* aspect of our beauty.

Lipstick does have a tendency to "catch" in dry patches on the lips. To achieve ultimate smoothness, lightly scrub your lips first with a little white sugar and a washcloth. If dryness persists, slick on a little lip primer to even out the texture before applying your lipstick for a satiny finish.

There's no rule for how to put on your lipstick—start up top or along the bottom, straight from the tube or using a lip brush. To make your color last longer, layer your lipstick. Slick on a first coat, blot with a tissue, and then add a second swipe for enduring loveliness.

To perfect your lippy look, trace the outside of your lipsticked lips with a little concealer, using light strokes with a small brush. This brings light to your mouth, creating a pillowy effect. Heavenly!

Sheer coral lip gloss complements all skin tones,
no matter what your age.

If your color bleeds when wearing gloss by itself,
simply trace the lips first with a clear lip liner.

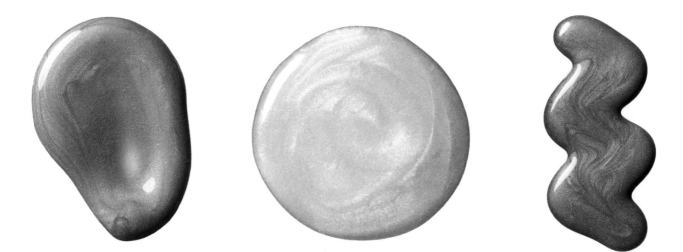

LIP GLOSS

Oh, lip gloss, how I adore thee. So many addictive shades. And, come on, how else can you sweep on sexy in seconds?

Lip gloss has a lot of pout perks. It's fast and easy, the shine accentuates your lip shape, and its dewiness looks modern, hip, and youthful. Wear it solo or over lipstick—just don't limit yourself. Today's glosses offer a huge range of looks from high-impact shine to subtle, moist sheen.

For optimum results, older women should choose a subdued gloss that offers a more opaque, dewy finish and skip the sticky vinyl-finish glosses. Younger ladies can go crazy with the maximum wet-slick look.

Although lip gloss works well on all lip shapes, it lives fast and dies young. You gotta gloss early and often. But it's oh so worth it!

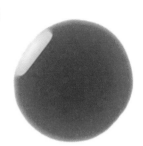

TINTED LIP BALMS AND STAINS

The new tinted lip balms are fantastic, especially for women who don't like the feel of lipstick or the stickiness of some glosses. Tinted lip balms give your lips that lively hint of color while moisturizing and protecting them at the same time.

Lip stains are another great option. Usually found in gel or liquid form, they stain the lips with a just-bitten color that stays all day. Because lip stains only offer color, I like to use a moisturizing tinted lip balm after applying them to give the lips the moisture they need and to double the color for a long-wearing look.

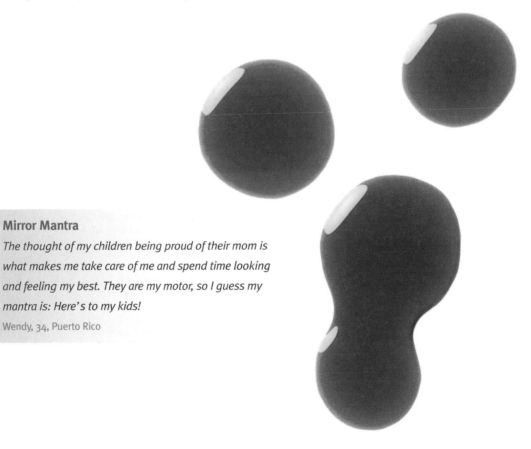

Mirror Mantra

The thought of my children being proud of their mom is what makes me take care of me and spend time looking and feeling my best. They are my motor, so I guess my mantra is: Here's to my kids!

Wendy, 34, Puerto Rico

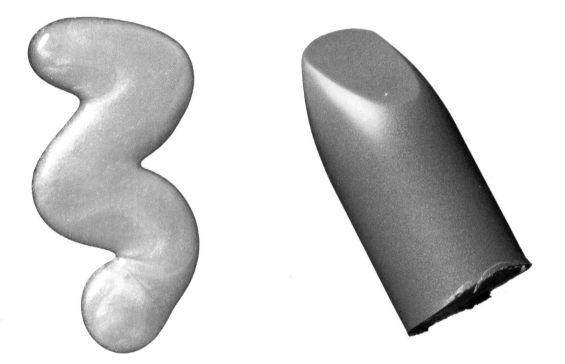

Play Up Your Pucker

If you have . . .

SMALL LIPS

Make the most of small lips by using light to midtone shades that contain a pearly shimmer. Start by highlighting the Cupid's bow (that little dip on the top lip) and under the lower lip with a bit of white highlight shimmer. This picks up light and frames the shape of your lips to make them stand out. Next, apply a light lip color that glows. Avoid really dark shades and matte finishes; they cause your sweet smile to recede.

You can also intensify your lips' impact by first applying a midtone lipstick with a hint of shimmer, then adding a dab of sparkling lip gloss to the center of the lower lip.

If you want to play with reds or deeper hues, go for sheer lipsticks, glosses, or tinted balms for a chic slash of color!

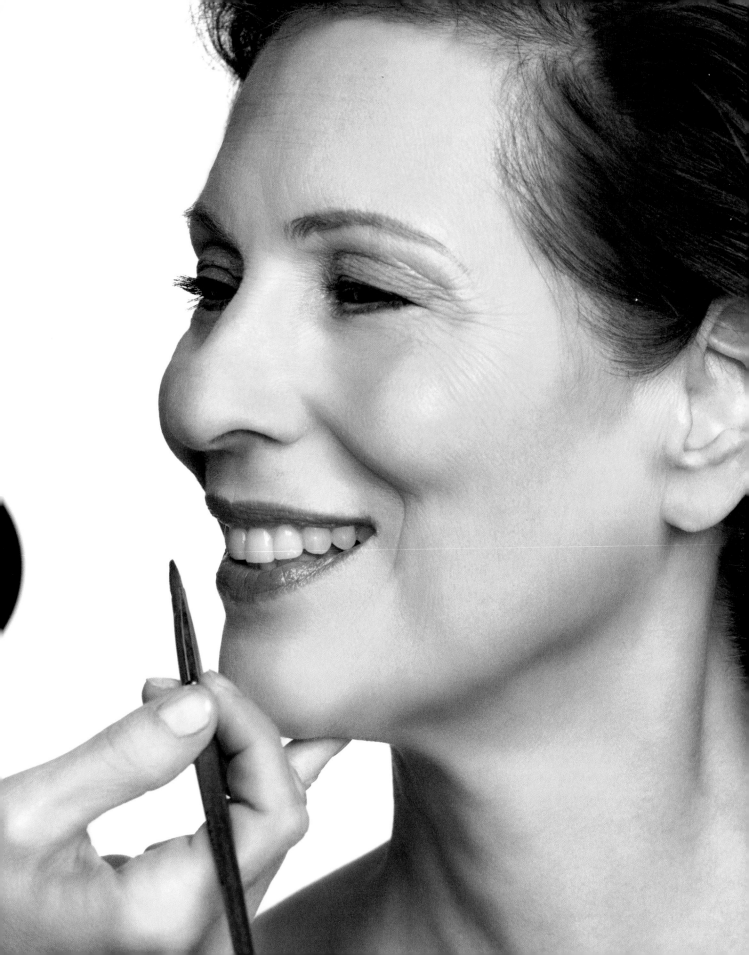

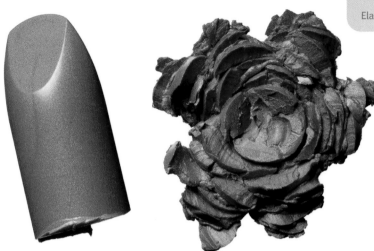

MEDIUM LIPS

Medium-size lips come alive when embellished with color. Check out bright and bold shades for evening drama or romantic and natural hues for daytime.

You can always apply lipstick in a bright shade, then tone it down by sweeping on a lighter gloss on top.

Medium-lipped ladies can pull off a classic red lipstick with ease, so go for it!

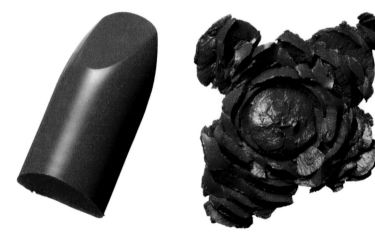

LARGE LIPS

Bold, daring colors look divine on bountiful lips, especially when paired with minimal makeup elsewhere. Skip high-shine lip glosses, as they can appear goopy on larger lips. Instead, head for satin or creamy matte-finish lipsticks, moist-looking glosses, and tinted balms. Yummy!

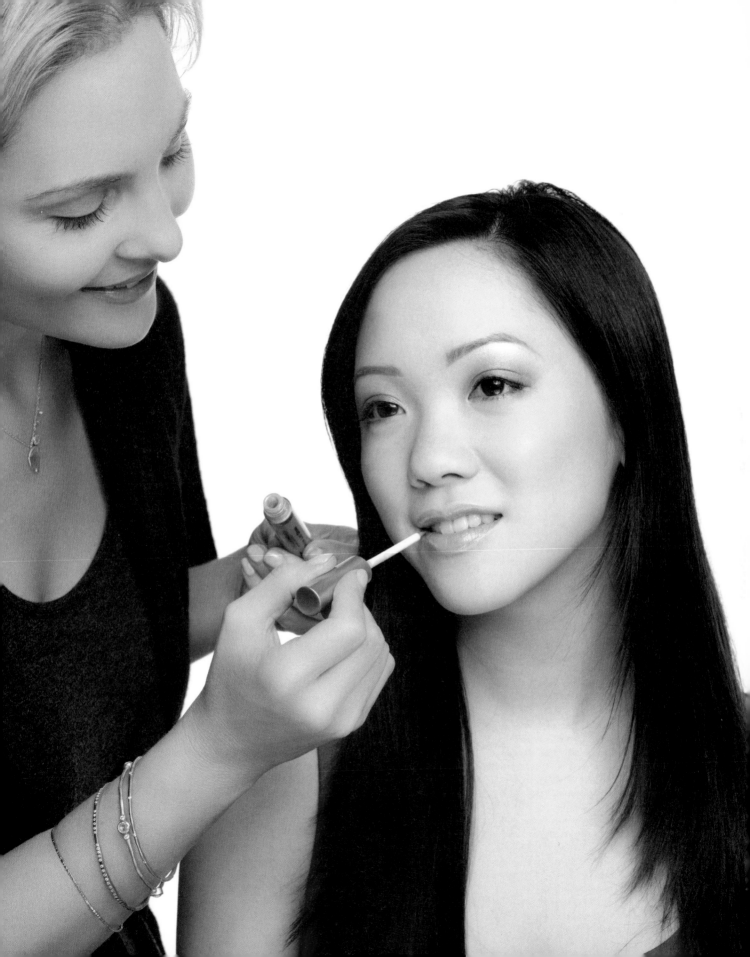

Spread Something Wonderful:
Contagious Compliments

Isn't a smile the best accessory ever? It's free. It's easy. It matches any outfit!

Only one thing can improve upon a happy grin–bringing a smile to another person's face by paying a sincere compliment.

We've been talking a lot about stopping negativity in its tracks and taking a positive approach to our beauty. But it doesn't end there, my friend. To truly unleash our beauty revolution, we must spread the goodness around by praising the beauty of our sisters.

Too often we admire from afar, or worse, let envy override our better nature. Either way, we stay silent and miss out on the opportunity to cultivate more joyful, positive energy in the world. Let's not let another chance slip from our grasp.

Let's start spreading something wonderful–compliments. They are positively contagious, and I say, bring on the epidemic!

If you see something lovely about a woman or young girl, *say something*! Complimenting clothing is an easy start. But if you want to really lift a lady's spirit, speak your praises about something she offers with her natural beauty, creative intelligence, and kindness.

*I noticed how patient you are with your daughter. I hope to be as good
a mother myself someday.*

Your eyes look so sparkling and bright today.

That smart idea of yours really got me thinking. Thanks for the inspiration!

You have the most gorgeous skin!

Whether she's a friend, a coworker, a stranger, a family member, or a regular rider on your morning train, every woman deserves to be noticed and noted for her unique goodness. When you speak up, you "up" her day and yours. What could be better? Let's get on it!

Carmindy Fan Q&A

Q: *I love my full lips, and I'm a gloss girl. What can I do to keep it from migrating if I'm not a pencil person?*

—Erika, 32, Orlando, FL

A: The trick is to line your lips with a clear lip liner. This colorless liner will seal in the gloss with an invisible waxy barrier, so you'll never have that ring-around-the-mouth look.

Q: *How do I use makeup so that people will see my smile and not my braces (which are coming off in a few months)?*

—Kim, 26, Mississauga, ON

A: Choose a rich, hydrating lipstick in a floral shade, but skip the shimmer. Anything super shiny or sparkly will accentuate the gleam of the braces. A moisturizing color will make your lips look luscious and your smile contagious.

Q: *The hairs on my upper lip seem to be more noticeable as I get older. How can I remove them so the focus stays on my full lips?*

—Anna, 39, Nashville, TN

A: For the sensitive upper lip area, I recommend a quick, inexpensive waxing at the local salon. It's not painless, but it's fast and will keep those hairs at bay.

Q: *I prefer a simple, outdoorsy look but want to try a little color. What should I try?*

—Katrina, 25, Cheyenne, WY

A: You are the perfect candidate for tinted lip balms. They offer moisture and protection with a pop of light, sheer color.

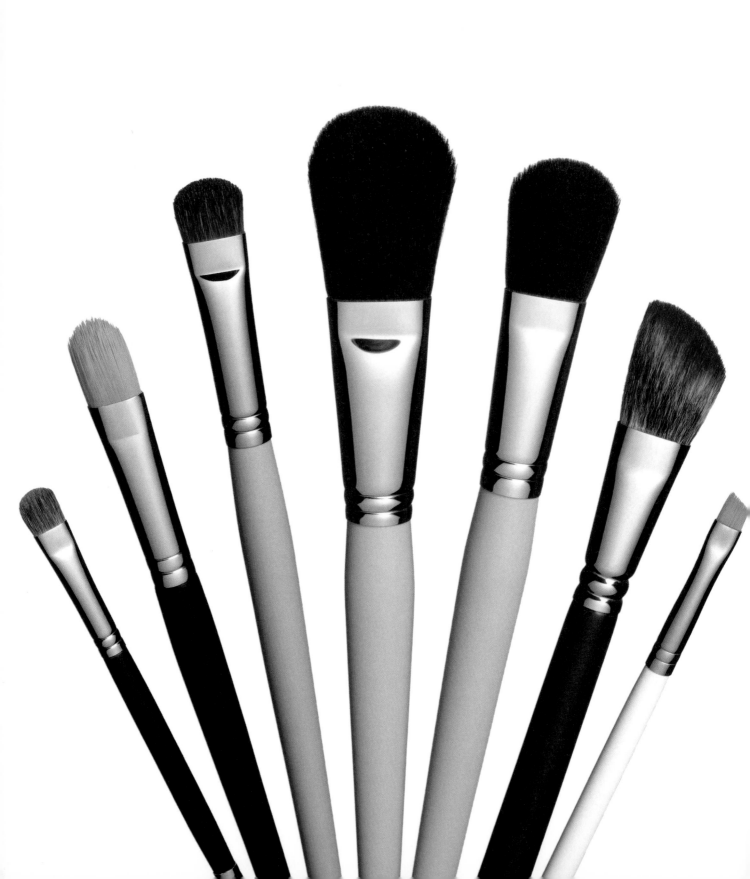

Only as you know yourself can your brain serve you as a sharp and efficient tool.

—BERNARD BARUCH

chapter nine *tool* time

We wouldn't expect a chef to create a gourmet feast with only a spoon and a paring knife. Nor would we hand Michelangelo a toothbrush and await the Sistine Chapel. Yet when it comes to makeup, most of us do without the tools that can make the difference between satisfactory and stunning results.

You've already learned how to use the right products in the right places to achieve your best look. Using the right tools will make flawless application a breeze and can actually streamline your daily routine. Believe it.

That said, there's absolutely no need to run out and buy *everything* you see here. Start with the items that help enhance your feature focus, and build your toolbox as you continue to experiment. Enjoy your beauty journey, sugar!

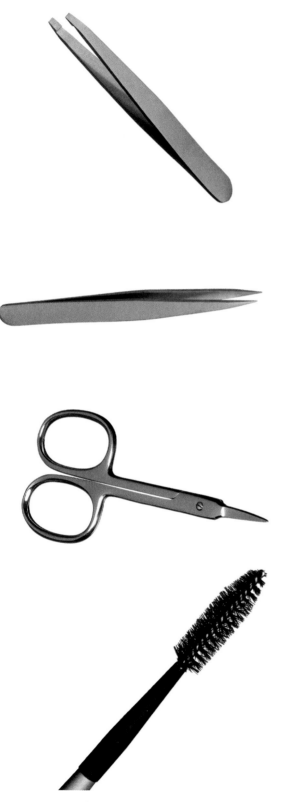

My Must-Have Tools

SLANTED-EDGE TWEEZERS

If you've let your brows go wild for a while, use slanted-edge tweezers to easily pull out thick-rooted or long brows. They grab more than one hair at a time, so take it slow.

POINTED-EDGE TWEEZERS

So precise you could do heart surgery with these babies. They're also great for fine-tuning a brow line, as they grab the tiny hairs that slanted tweezers can't handle. Use your pointies every couple of days, and you'll stay perfectly groomed.

SCISSORS

Cuticle scissors are ideal for trimming extra-long eyebrows and snipping false lashes in half when creating a sexy, dramatic eye look.

BROW BRUSH

This spooley little tool is perfect for brushing up your brows so you can snip away any long strays. It also grooms your arches into super shape.

ANGLED BROW BRUSH

Choose a flat-angled brush that's very stiff; it will feather on the little bit of brow color needed to enhance your natural brow hairs.

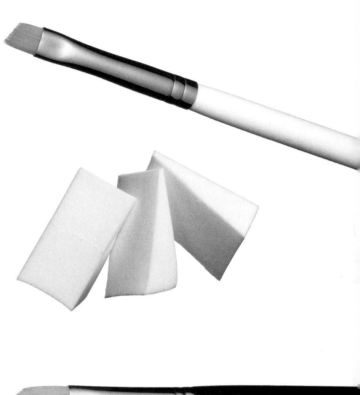

NONLATEX SPONGES

Look closely before you buy. The best nonlatex sponges have no visible pores. Porous sponges suck up foundation, leave streaks, and crumble quickly. Nonporous sponges simply smooth on foundation, allowing you to buff and polish your complexion to perfection.

UNDER-EYE CONCEALER BRUSH

I love this synthetic half-dome brush; it blends on brightening concealer with ease, creating an energized, wide-awake look.

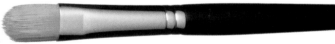

SMALL-TIPPED CONCEALER BRUSH

This baby is the perfect size for blending foundation, concealer, or a mixture of both right onto any trouble spots. A little dab will do ya—so this brush saves you time and product.

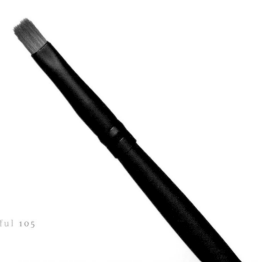

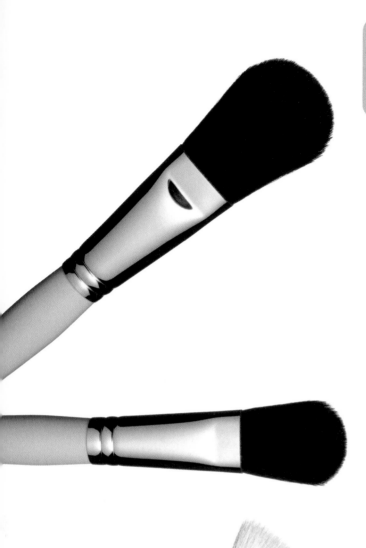

POWDER AND BLUSH BRUSHES

Switcheroo time. In the old days, we used small blush brushes that picked up too much color for small cheek areas. (Remember red-slashed eighties cheeks?) And we used a large, fluffy powder brush to cover our skin with heavy matte loose powder, erasing our complexions in the dust storm!

Today we want a natural blush flush and skin we can actually see. So swap 'em. The smaller brush is best for applying face powder to areas that need it, leaving the rest dewy fresh. The big fluffy brush is best for blush, as it hugs the apples of the cheeks, creating a soft, natural rosiness. Got it? Good!

FAN BRUSH

Use this funny-looking brush to apply powder highlighter to the tops of the cheekbones. Keep yours soft and fluffy so it delivers the perfect pop of shimmer.

BRONZER BRUSH

Sister to powder brushes, a bronzer brush has a slightly angled shape to sweep sunshine to the temples, along the cheekbones, and on any other areas seeking a golden glow.

DOUBLE-ENDED HIGHLIGHTER BRUSH

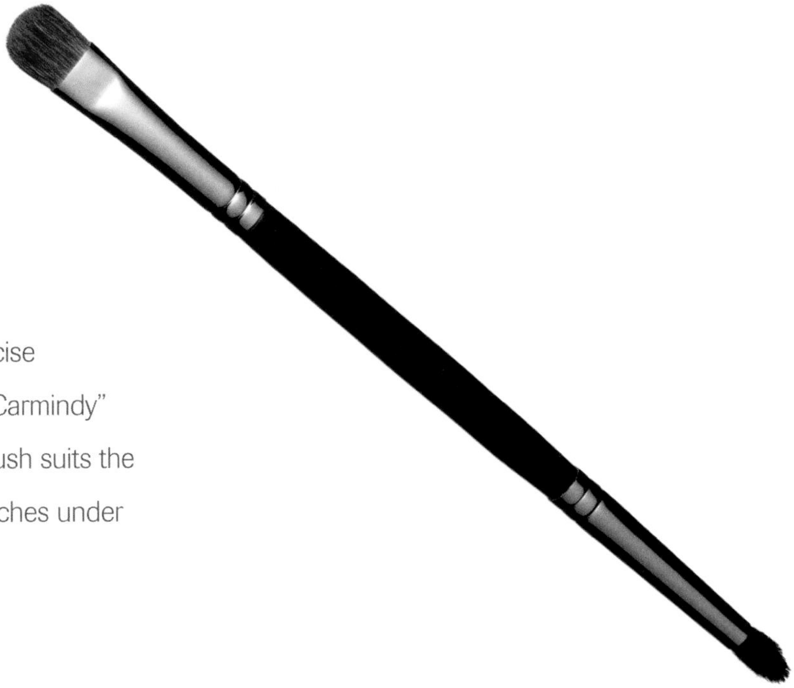

This two-for-one brush is perfect for the precise application of powdered highlighter to key "Carmindy" areas around your eyes. The small-tipped brush suits the inner corners of the eyes; the larger side reaches under the brow with ease.

ANGLED EYELINER BRUSH

Similar to the angled brow brush but with softer bristles, the eyeliner brush gently glides on liner. Use it to smudge pencil or powdered eye shadow on the top or bottom lashes for a subtle effect, or dip the brush into cream or liquid liner for a more defined look.

LIQUID TRANSFORMER

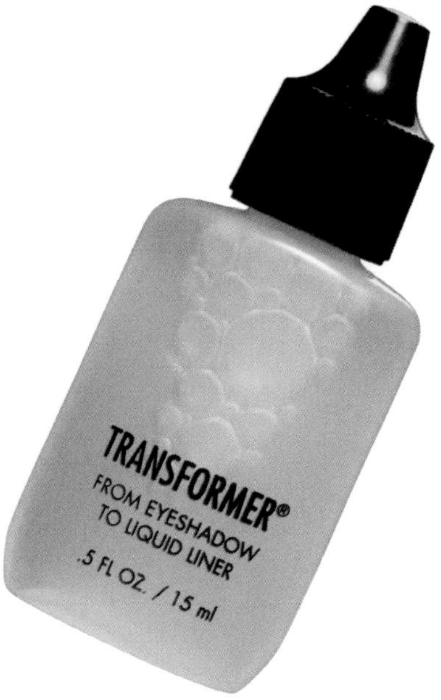

This clear liquid allows you to transform any eye shadow into a liquid liner. It's a great tool for experimenting with new eye looks. Simply put a drop on the back of your hand and drag your angled eyeliner brush through it. Then dip the brush into your favorite eye shadow, and apply it along the lash line.

TRANSFORMER®
FROM EYESHADOW
TO LIQUID LINER
.5 FL OZ. / 15 ml

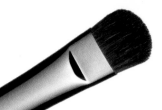

LID EYE SHADOW BRUSH

Whether playing with a smoky evening eye or applying a sheer wash of color for day, this eye shadow brush is the perfect size to sweep color onto your eyelid.

CREASE EYE SHADOW BRUSH

The crease area of the eye looks sculpted and smooth when you us this perfect-size brush. It lays on color softly, making blending a snap.

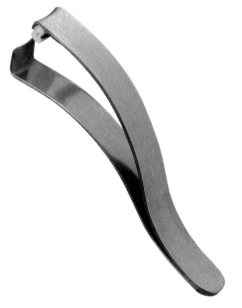

CORNER LASH CURLER

All lash curlers are not created equal. Traditional curlers don't fit many eye shapes and can leave chunks of lashes uncurled. A more effective, modern tool is the corner lash curler. It grips lashes section by section, offering better control. So whether you want a full fringe of perfectly curled lashes or flirty "wings" only at the outer edges, a corner lash curler is the way to go.

METAL LASH COMB

Oh, the horror stories I hear about women using needles and safety pins to separate their lashes. Yikes! What if your kid runs up behind you or you sneeze? Don't be foolish! Buy a metal lash comb to separate any clumps after you apply mascara. Remember to comb quickly—before the mascara dries—so you don't pull out any precious plumes.

LIP BRUSH

Most tinted lip balms and glosses with wands work fine on their own, but if you want a precisely painted lip, bust out your lip brush. I usually use mine to slick on a great evening lipstick.

SHARPENER

For eye and lip pencils, it's best to invest in a double-size sharpener. Regular pencils swirl in the smaller opening, fatter pencils in the larger one.

BLOTTING PAPERS

A pack of oil-absorbing blotting papers will keep shine in check and eliminate the need for constant repowdering.

Carmindy Fan Q&A

Q: *I get so confused when it comes to lining the eye with a brush. Any advice?*

—Jessica, 26, Lake Villa, IL

A: Go for a flat, thin, angular brush. Choose one with natural bristles for a finer blend, and use it to apply powder eye shadow as liner or to apply cake, cream, or gel liner formulas. For liquid eyeliner, dab some on the back of your hand and drag the angle brush through it. That's how we professionals create those perfect sweeps. If you mess up along the way, use a small-tipped concealer brush with a bit of foundation or concealer on it to erase any wayward streaks.

Q: *I apply liquid foundation with cosmetic sponges and find it really covers my dark circles. Applying make-up with my fingers never worked as well. Do you agree?*

—Carolyn, 56, Birmingham, AL

A: It's truly a matter of personal preference. I apply my foundation with my fingers, then lightly buff it to a flawless finish with a nonlatex sponge. I then spot-conceal using a brush. But if sponges work best for you, go for it.

Q: *How sharp should my eyeliner pencil be?*

—Jessica, 30, Aurora, IL

A: Very sharp for precision application. If you want a smudgier look, roll the tip between clean fingers so it's a little rounder. Remember to sharpen pencils before each use to keep bacteria at bay and ease your application.

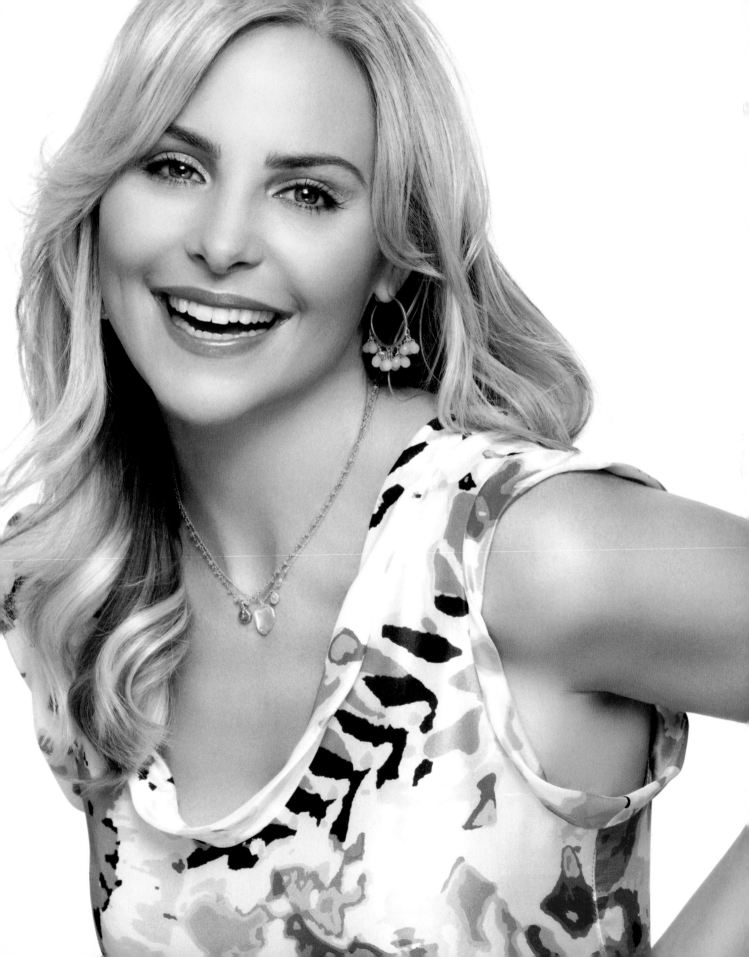

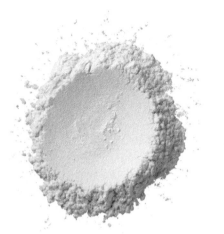
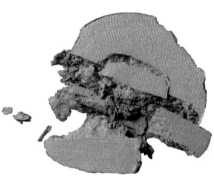
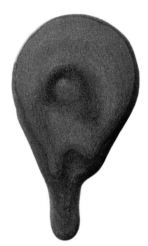
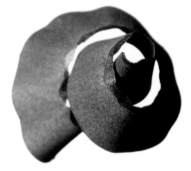
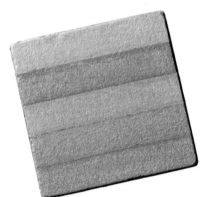
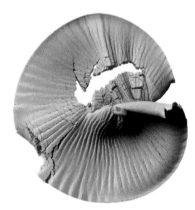
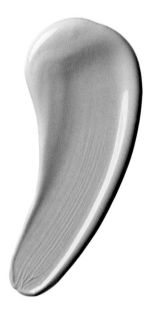
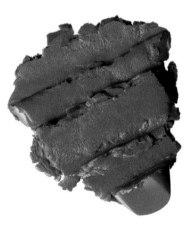
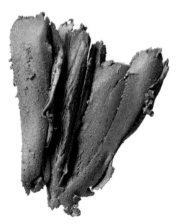

Though we travel the world over to find the beautiful,
we must carry it with us or we find it not.
—RALPH WALDO EMERSON

chapter ten ## what's in your makeup bag?

Every woman's collection of cosmetics and fragrances is a secret treasure chest containing her deepest beauty desires. Some products even hold special memories. That perfume you wore the night you met him. That lipstick that turned you into a disco diva. Those fluttery fake lashes that were the hit of the bachelorette party.

Clearly what's in your makeup bag says a lot about you. Many of us want to keep and carry everything with us at all times. We need to fight that feeling and lighten our load!

Getting positively beautiful means getting real with who you are and what you need *today*. Parting with the past can be painful, but it is always liberating. Could clearing out your beauty clutter be the start of something even bigger? You bet.

Step onboard my streamline express to look stunning at home and on the go!

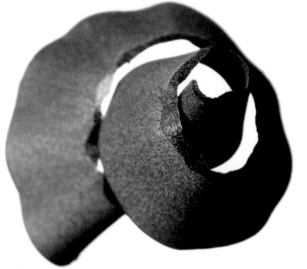

Confronting the Chaos

Most women perform some form of spring cleaning on our homes and weed through our wardrobes as the seasons change. But how often do we clear out our makeup bags and drawers? Yep. Busted!

When I do private consultations, I get an inside look at women's cosmetic stockpiles. Let me tell ya, it ain't pretty. Picture if you will Ms. Carmindy attempting to keep a smile on my face as I gaze in horror at a filthy, ancient, oozing pile of products.

What do I often discover? Broken eye shadows, a nub of an eyeliner, some dried-out mascara, a favorite lipstick gouged deeply from sticking a lip brush in it, a prehistoric cotton swab coated in nastiness, a hair band, dull and cheap tweezers, a blush brush flattened and rubbed down to a Brillolike roughness, crumbling sponges, and dried pieces of gum so hard you can snap 'em in half. Sound familiar, ladies?

Now's not the time for feeling guilty; instead, get busy! Take everything—yes, everything—out of your drawers, cabinets, and cubbyholes to start the sort-and-purge process.

Humid bathroom conditions breed bacteria, so first clean and disinfect all your storage areas. While everything is drying out, spread out your beauty products on a table for examination and elimination.

Old makeup and dirty tools can harbor bacteria, leading to infections and breakouts. Here are my expiration dates for beauty basics:

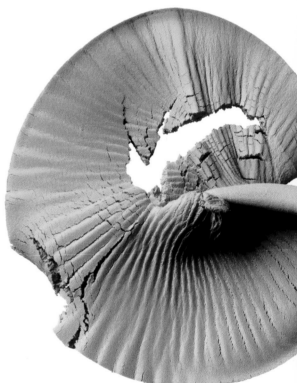

- Foundation: 1 year

- Concealer: 1 year

- Face powder: 1 year

- Powder blush or bronzer: 1 year

- Cream blush or bronzer: 1 year

- Mascara: 6 months

- Eyeliner: 2 years, but sharpen pencils frequently

- Liquid eyeliner: 6 months

- Eye shadow: 1 year

- Lipstick: 2 years

- Brushes: wash weekly

- Sponges: wash weekly; replace monthly

Above and beyond these rules, do any of your products smell or look funky? Toss 'em. Find anything you haven't used in a year? Ditch it. Make room for what works for you *today*. Treat yourself to a few new products and modern shades.

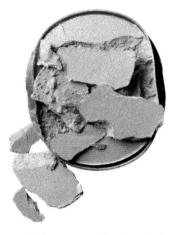

To keep your budget in line, consider rejuvenating worn-down (but not worn-out) makeup. Here are a few tricks:

- If you have favorite lipsticks that are whittled down, scoop out what's left and put each shade in a little plastic pillbox for a great palette of lip colors to mix and match.
- If some of your pressed eye shadows are broken, turn them into loose shadows by storing them in clear film-roll canisters.
- Dried-out, crusty mascara can be reliquefied by running the sealed tube under hot water for five minutes. However, please heed the 6-month replacement rule on mascara; swollen, infected eyes are *not hot.*

Now that you've got your home beauty bar whisked clean and well stocked, let's attack how to pack up for on-the-go gorgeousness.

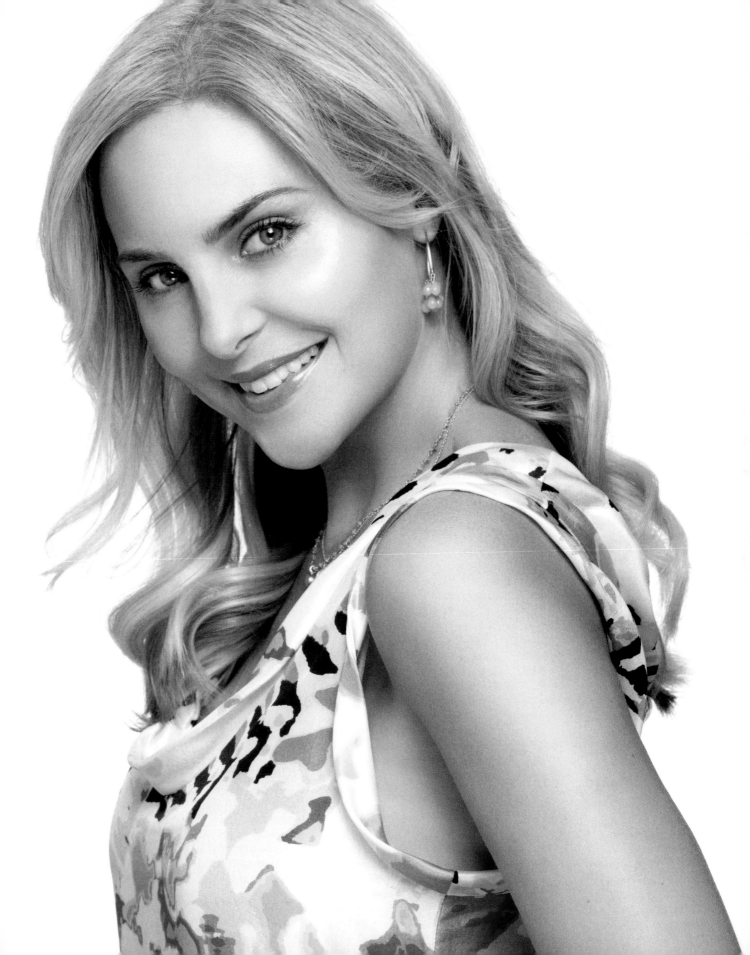

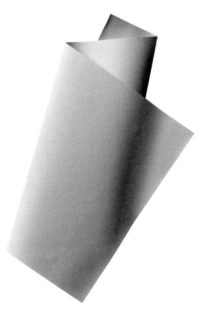

PURSE

Here's a test: Shake your purse for a second. Is that the sound of a million products I hear rattling around the bottom? Time to get organized, dearie!

If you've properly applied your makeup at home, there's no need to carry around your entire bathroom. All of your touching-up tackle should fit nicely into a small, clean cosmetics bag and should be slipped into your tote.

First and foremost, you need a mirrored compact face powder. It's great to take a moment in the middle of a hectic day to pause and appreciate your femininity. Take hold of that compact, gaze at yourself lovingly, and repeat your mirror mantra while powdering any shiny spots.

You know I'm not fond of all-day lip products, so keep your tinted lip balm, lipstick, or gloss at the ready. Slick on a fresh pop of color after coffee breaks and meals.

Cotton swabs are a must for cleaning up smudges or smears, and blotting papers are great for zapping any excess shine before you powder.

That's it! You're now so sleek, you may want to shop for a smaller, more chic bag!

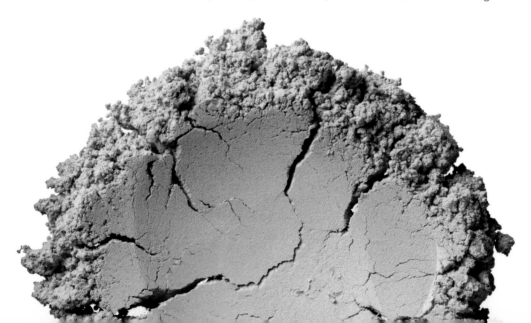

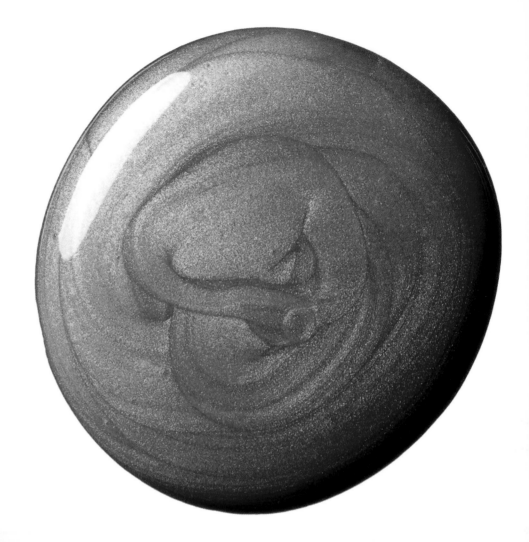

Table Tricks

A shout-out to Emily Post and my grandmother: It's poor form to touch up your makeup while at the dining table. If you need to redo your lipstick or powder your nose, please do so in the *powder room*.

That said, I admit I don't always follow Grandma's advice. I'm a lippy sneak, and you can join my tribe. Secretly remove your lip color from your bag under the table, and dab a bit onto your pinky finger. Casually put your elbow on the table and bring your hand up to your chin, listening intently to the conversation. Now start to subtly tap your lips with that potent pinky as you nod to whatever's being said. People won't notice a thing except your charming smile.

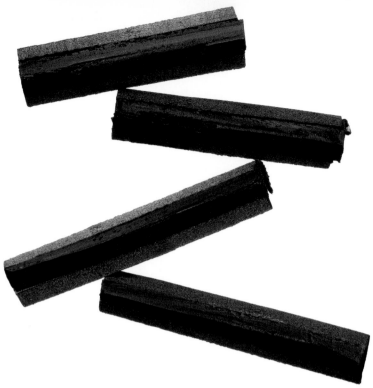

DESK

I believe we make our own luck in life. Someone once defined luck as what happens when opportunity meets preparation. You never know when a great job lead or after-work party invitation might arrive, so be ready to get lucky by stashing a little makeup bag in your desk.

Your office beauty supplies should include:

- blotting papers

- a bottle of foundation and a small-tipped concealer brush

- blush and a blush brush

- dark eyeliner and a cotton swab

- a midtone or contour eye shadow and an eye shadow brush

- a highlighter powder and an eye shadow brush to apply it

- day and evening shades of lipstick or gloss

- a powder compact

- your favorite perfume

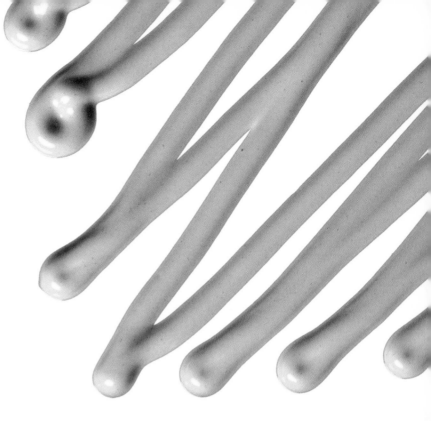

When the whistle blows, you can go from polished professional to nightlife lovely in seconds with just a few adjustments to your day face. Here's how:

Step 1: First, use the blotting papers to eliminate any accumulated shine.

Step 2: Next, dip your small-tipped concealer brush into a little foundation and touch up any trouble spots on your skin. (You don't want to blend on a whole new face of foundation, because it will just look heavy and masklike.)

Step 3: Dust on a little face powder.

Step 4: Play up your eyes by smudging dark eyeliner along the lash line. This gives you a thicker-looking lash line without adding a clumpy load of extra mascara.

Step 5: Sweep on your evening eye shadow and place highlighting powder on the brow bone, the inside corners of the eyes, and your décolletage.

Step 6: Swirl on a little more blush.

Step 7: Add on your evening shade of lip color.

Step 8: Spritz on a sexy scent, and you're ready to knock 'em dead!

TRAVEL

Traveling is one of the greatest joys in my life and is a true blessing of my profession. From Milan's busy streets to tiny villages in Tanzania, hitting the road and observing this world's wondrous cultural diversity has really shaped who I am. Even better, I've been privileged to meet beautiful women on every trip. They've cemented my belief that there is no set "ideal" except being beautifully who we are. What an inspiration!

The challenge in all this jet-setting is choosing what to pack to avoid looking haggard without being bogged down along the way. I believe in a less-is-more approach. A journey is a great opportunity to scale back your regimen and free up time to experience more of your adventure. Today's airport regulations are actually helpful, as you simply *can't* take everything with you.

Your best travel beauty buddy is a 1-quart Ziploc bag. Ms. Ziploc instills discipline! To avoid seeing a TSA agent trash your precious cosmetics cargo, keep any liquids/gels to three ounces or less. This does not mean you can take the three ounces of moisturizer left in a five-ounce bottle. The packaging must be marked as three ounces or less.

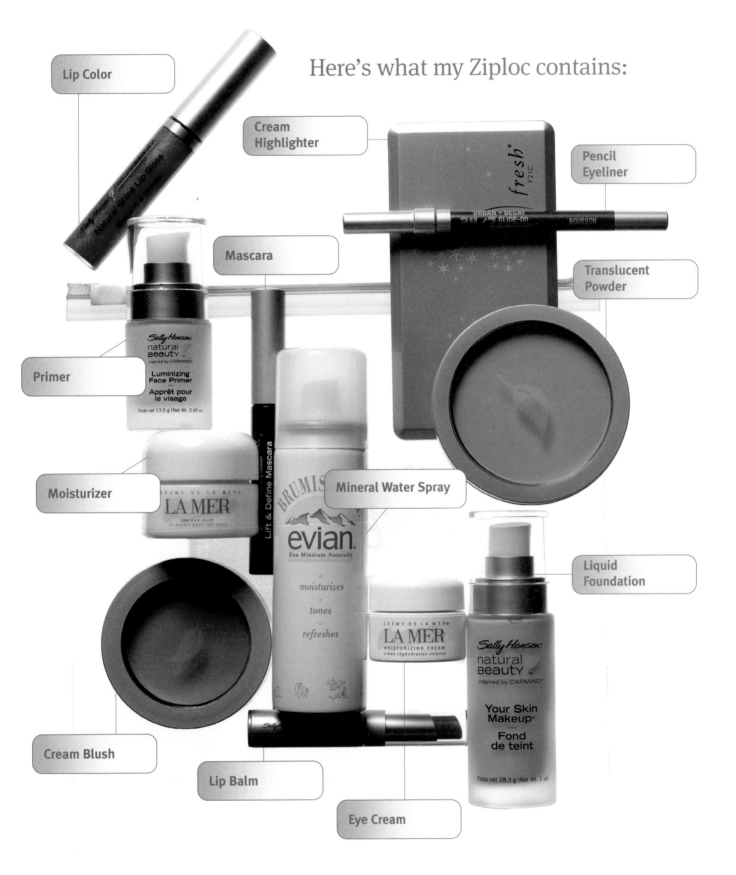

Here's what my Ziploc contains:

Lip Color

Cream Highlighter

Pencil Eyeliner

Mascara

Translucent Powder

Primer

Moisturizer

Mineral Water Spray

Liquid Foundation

Cream Blush

Lip Balm

Eye Cream

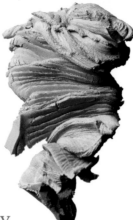

PLANE PRETTY

When traveling by plane, you need to protect your skin from the drying effects of a pressurized air cabin. I like to begin my trip with a bare face that has been slathered with a good moisturizer. Once you are comfortably in the air, apply a great lip balm for a sweet smile that won't look parched. Tap on a little eye cream or a rich moisturizer around the delicate eye area. I use the free samples offered at many department stores.

While onboard, avoid consuming alcohol and salty snacks, which can exacerbate dehydration. Instead, drink lots of water and bring your own nibbles, like fresh fruit, unsalted nuts, and baby carrots. I also try to spritz a little mineral water on my face during the flight. (I recommend doing this in the lavatory so you don't shower your fellow travelers!)

Shortly before landing, put down that tray table and whip out your 5-minute face supplies to guarantee a gorgeous arrival. (PS: Window seats offer the best lighting.)

My 5-minute face technique is perfect for your entire trip.

- First, apply primer and a liquid foundation.
- Follow with a creamy blush on the apples of your cheeks and a dab of cream highlighter under your brows, on the inside corners of your eyes, and on top of your cheekbones.
- Next, dust on a light translucent powder and line the upper lash line with a pencil.
- Finish with mascara on the upper lashes and a slick of your favorite lip color.

Voilà: A fresh appearance sure to have the customs agents swooning!

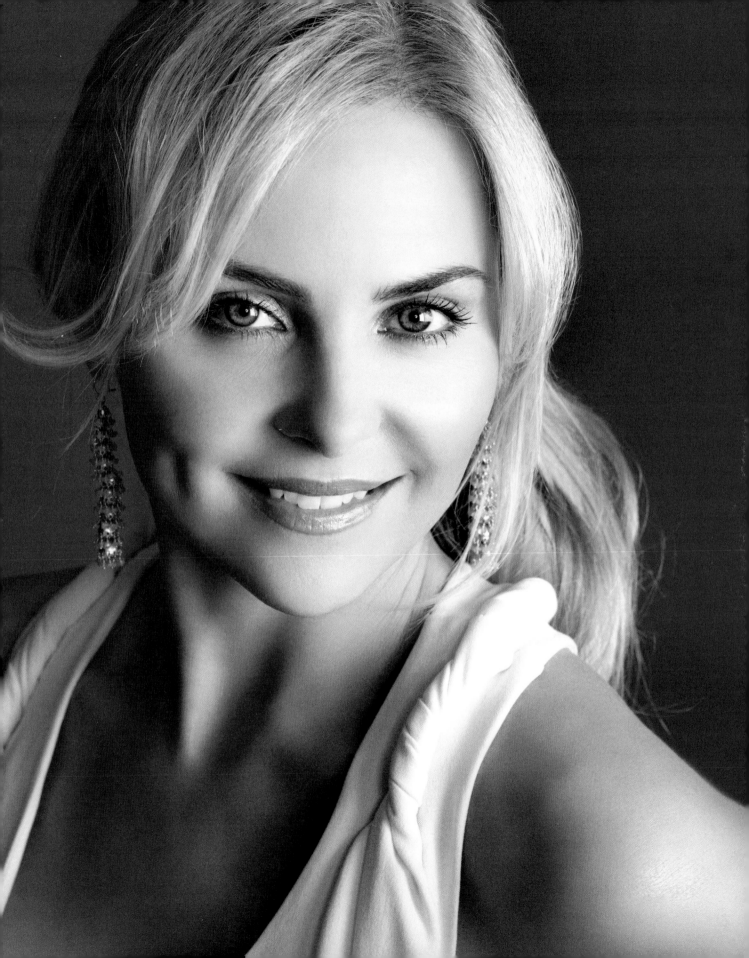

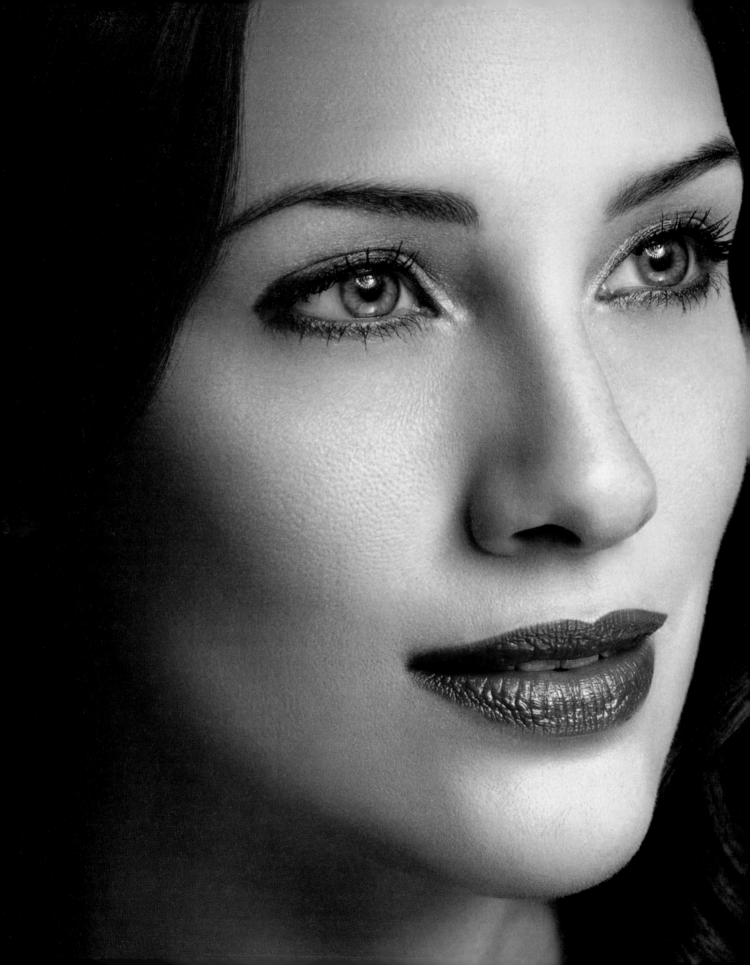

One touch of nature makes the whole world kin.

—WILLIAM SHAKESPEARE

chapter eleven beauty for every season

Mother Nature is one fascinating babe, and boy does she have a way of keeping us on our toes! Whether the mercury is climbing or *brrrrrr*, in comes that first chilling wind, our beauty routines need to change right along with the seasons.

When it's time to "spring forward" or "fall back" and reset your clocks, it's also a great time to reevaluate your approach to makeup and skin care for the coming months. Switching to products that work with the weather will help keep you looking fresh and gorgeous. And, taking cues from Mother Nature, you should also change up color choices a bit to stay current and at the top of your game.

Follow these tips, and I can guarantee this beauty forecast: *fabulous!*

Spring and Summer

Heat and humidity can make keeping makeup in place a real challenge. As we perspire to stay cool, we also fire up the skin's sebum glands, creating an oilier complexion. Our handiwork tends to melt right off. However, there are lots of ways to stay as vibrant as a summer sunrise all day—and look as hot!

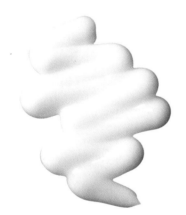

SKIN

First and foremost, sunscreen will save you! It's an absolute *must*, no matter the season. Call me Mama Carmindy, but you should be as religious about applying sunscreen as you are about brushing your teeth. Apply sunscreen right after you moisturize, or purchase a moisturizer that has sunscreen built right in. You will help avoid premature aging, skin cancer, and wrinkles. Protect yourself now; pour on that magic prevention potion every day.

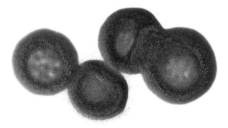

SELF-TANNER

If you still desire a glowing beach-babe look, choose one of the many self-tanners on the market. Some formulas gradually build up to the perfect shade; others make you savage overnight. So experiment to find the one that suits your skin and doesn't leave you looking orange or unnaturally tan. Tanorexia is tacky!

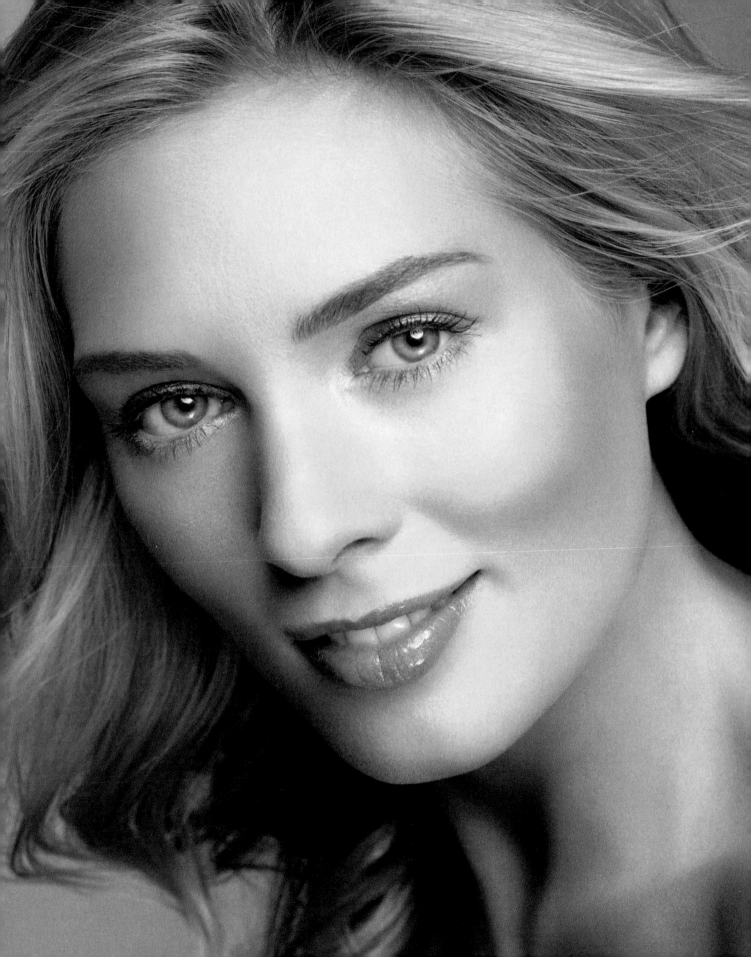

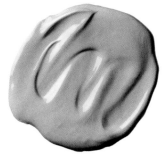

FOUNDATION

You don't have to change your foundation every season; stick with the one that works best for you. To control surges of shine, use a primer or mattifying gel before foundation to keep your face fresh. If you use a self-tanner, you may want to buy a "summer" bottle of your foundation that's one shade darker to match the tanner you. If you like the feel of lighter, more sheer coverage, try a tinted moisturizer with built-in sunscreen. Its texture is the most comfortable in extreme heat.

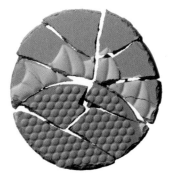

BRONZER

Want a little summer sun without having to go all out with a self-tanner? Pick up a powder or spray bronzer to give your skin a temporary kiss of color that will stay put and look natural.

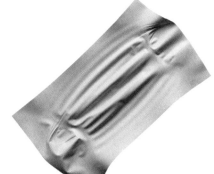

OIL CONTROL

Steamy conditions can cause even the driest complexion to get a bit greasy. To stay glowy, not goopy, pack your purse with blotting papers. I always blot first to absorb excess oil, and then apply a sheer powder to control the shine. If you just add powder on top of the slick spots, you may wind up with a thick, cakey mess. Keep a clean, healthy look and blot, babycakes!

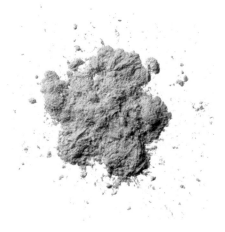

EYES

For your eye makeup, stick with powder-formula highlighters and eye shadows. Using sheer powders ensures longevity, with color that won't fade or get creasy. Choose waterproof gel pencil eyeliners, waterproof liquid eyeliners, and waterproof or tube technology mascaras. When the heat is on, these stay-put products guarantee a long-lasting look even after a dip in the pool.

CHEEKS

For cheeks, pick powder-formula blushes for a soft look and cheek stains or gels for a natural-looking, sweatproof flush. Any type of cream formula makeup will likely melt right off your face. They look nice and sheer when they go on, but they'll do a disappearing act on you.

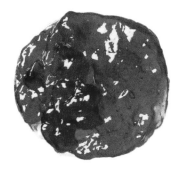

LIPS

Lips look their best with tinted lip balms that offer color and comfort or with sheer lip glosses in the brightest, juiciest colors. When you're switching up your wardrobe, be sure to update your lippy collection with hot, trendy shades of gloss. The sheer factor allows you to take chances with bold color for a hot new look. Sizzling!

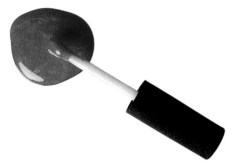

COLORS

Your whole approach to makeup should parallel how you pick your warm-weather outfits: namely, lighter and more carefree. And your color choices should mirror the blooming bounty of nature. For cheeks and lips, think floral or coral. For eyes and skin, bronze or golden shades look amazing.

Pastels and brights look great this time of year, too, but remember my watercolor painting idea and go for sheer shades that allow the skin to show through. Opaque shades are too heavy, like an oil painting. Stick with a hint of color, and you'll be a masterpiece!

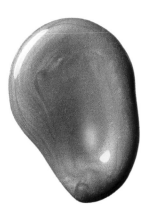

Fall and Winter

Chilly temperatures and dry air tend to send us all to Chapped City. The keys to relief are moisture and hydration. Though we're not as thirsty, drinking more water is a big boost for wintertime skin. Putting a humidifier in your bedroom adds a new dimension to beauty sleep. And switching to hydrating makeup formulas and richer moisturizers is a smart move.

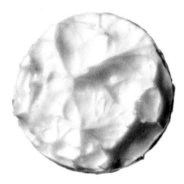

SKIN AND CHEEKS

Face Cream

Your nighttime skin care regimen needs to be stepped up a bit during these months. If you usually use a light lotion, switch to a heavier cream and add a rich eye cream to soften the fine lines that tend to be more prominent when skin is parched. Your eyes will thank you in the morning.

Primer

Applying a primer before foundation is crucial when the weather turns frigid. Primer helps eliminate dry patches and smooth out your skin's texture. Most formulas also contain light-reflecting particles that add a glowing radiance to brighten your complexion on even the darkest days of winter.

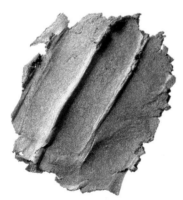

Highlighter

After applying foundation, choose cream or liquid highlighters for the tops of cheekbones to give your skin the dewy look it deserves. Swirl on cream blushes to bring life and color to your cheeks. Creamy formulas look and feel especially supple this time of year, so give them a go.

Powder

With face powder, use a very light hand to avoid a dry and chalky look. Ladies with very dry skin may want to skip it altogether. If you have oily skin, use a brush instead of a puff for a lighter finish.

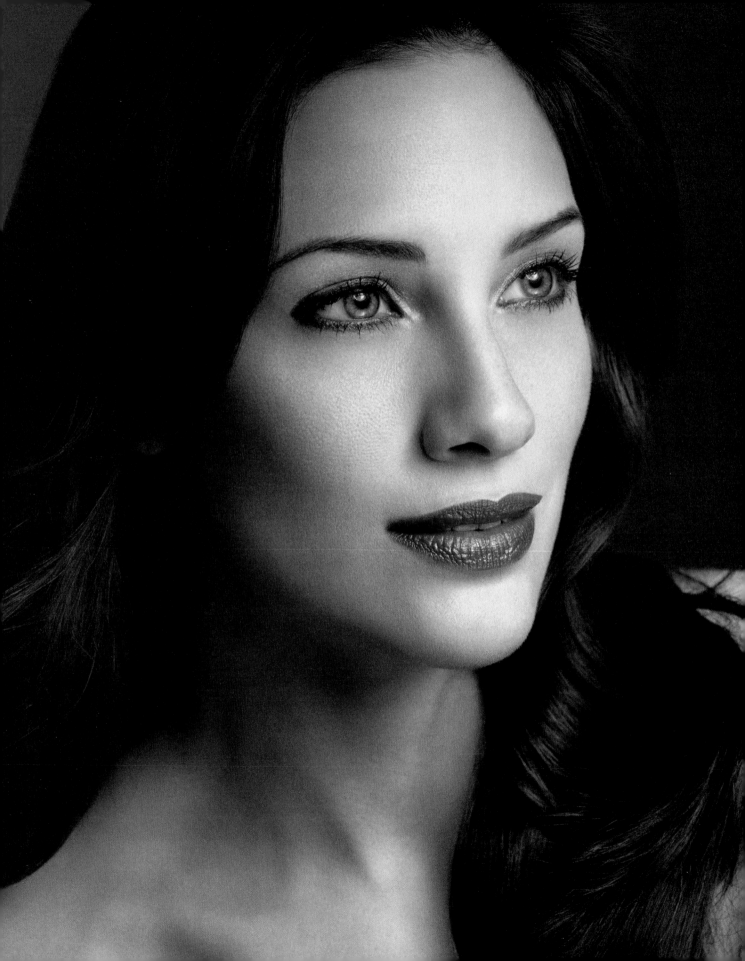

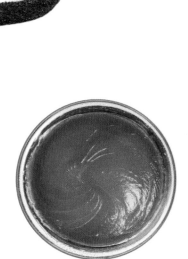

EYES

On the eyes, play with cream highlights and eye shadows that look smooth and satiny, not dry and crepey. For glide-on color that won't pull or tug, try one of the new gel pencil eyeliners for definition. For more drama, try sweeping on a line of liquid eyeliner, which looks fantastic against winter skin. Choose mascaras in regular or conditioning formulas so lashes stay lush in the cold, dry weather.

LIPS

Lips need extra TLC when it's freezing outside. I always keep a rich and creamy tinted lip balm in my purse for day and a nourishing, healing balm by my bedside for night. Constant vigilance combats evil dryness and keeps lips soft and smooth. Apply a moisturizing lipstick or gloss over your lip balm during the day to ensure chap-free lips that look as good as they feel.

COLORS

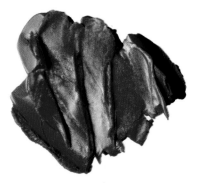

Color choices for fall and winter can be a bit more sensual and moody. For eyes, play with jewel tones or smoky, mysterious shades like silvery taupes or chocolate browns. For lips, try staining or painting them with berries, wines, or reds. Just pick your one feature focus, and power up the intensity. Smashing!

When holiday parties hit, get your fun and festive on. Rosy up those cheeks to bring warmth to paler skin, and play with false lashes, a bit of sparkle, or a reflective eye shadow for flirty flair. Your glorious presence will be the prettiest present ever!

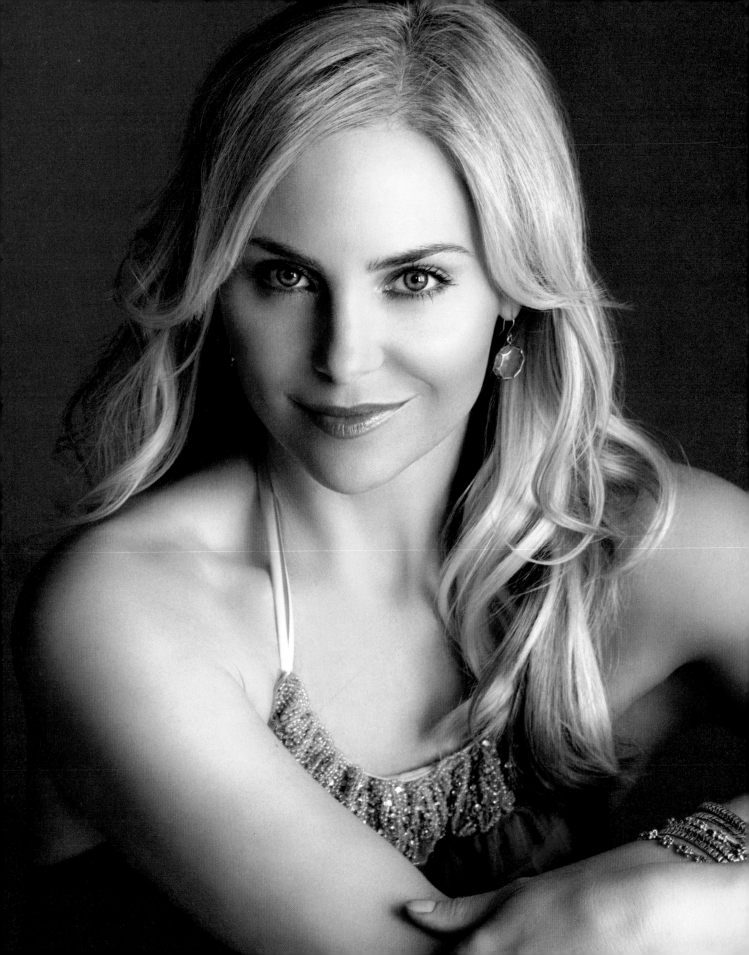

Carmindy Fan Q&A

Q: *How can I make my olive complexion look soft, dewy, and smooth in a dry climate?*

—Liz, 37, Denver, CO

A: Remember to exfoliate a few times a week to keep your skin smooth and polished. Use a good moisturizer in the morning and then follow with an application of primer. Next, smooth on a liquid foundation and choose cream-formula highlighter and blush. You may want to skip powder, as it may make your skin look drier. If you want to control shine, powder just the T-zone.

Q: *How should I moisturize my sensitive skin during the long Canadian winter?*

—Kathleen, 38, Ottawa, ON

A: Switch up your morning moisturizer from a lotion to a richer cream and apply a primer before smoothing on foundation. Apply powder sparingly so that most of your skin stays looking hydrated and fresh. Choose formulas that are paraben-free and filled with natural ingredients to keep sensitive skin happy.

Q: *I have seasonal allergies. How can I disguise morning puffiness and darkness around my eyes without applying heavy products that settle into fine lines?*

—Julie, 25, Denver, CO

A: Blasted allergies! So many of us suffer from them, but there are few remedies to ease the puffies.

- First, try a good nasal cleansing using a neti pot. Nasal irrigation is an ancient Ayurvedic practice from In-dia that helps your sinus cavities flush out nasty allergens, calming and soothing swollen areas. I have seen this work, and it's amazing.
- Get a good night's sleep, drink plenty of water, and do at least fifteen minutes of heart-pumping exercise each day. I know this is more than a quick tip, but trust me, cardio is the best beauty secret for puffy allergy eyes.
- Apply a foundation that's one shade darker to the swollen areas. Then, in the deeper crease, apply a brightening concealer to bring in a little light. Stay away from heavy concealers, and don't make yourself crazy trying to re-create your eyes. Instead, choose a fun lipstick color, and draw attention to your unstoppable grin.

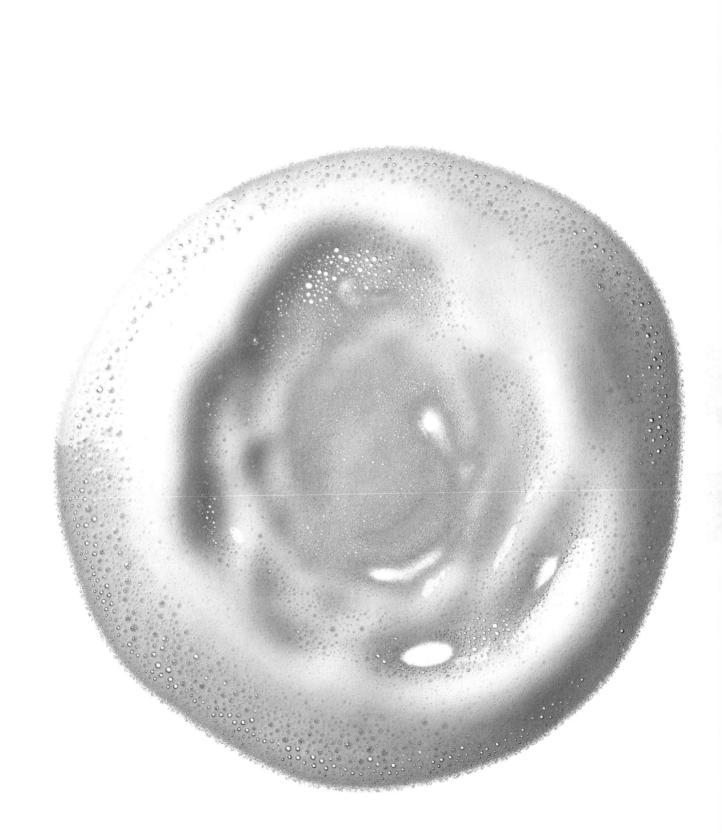

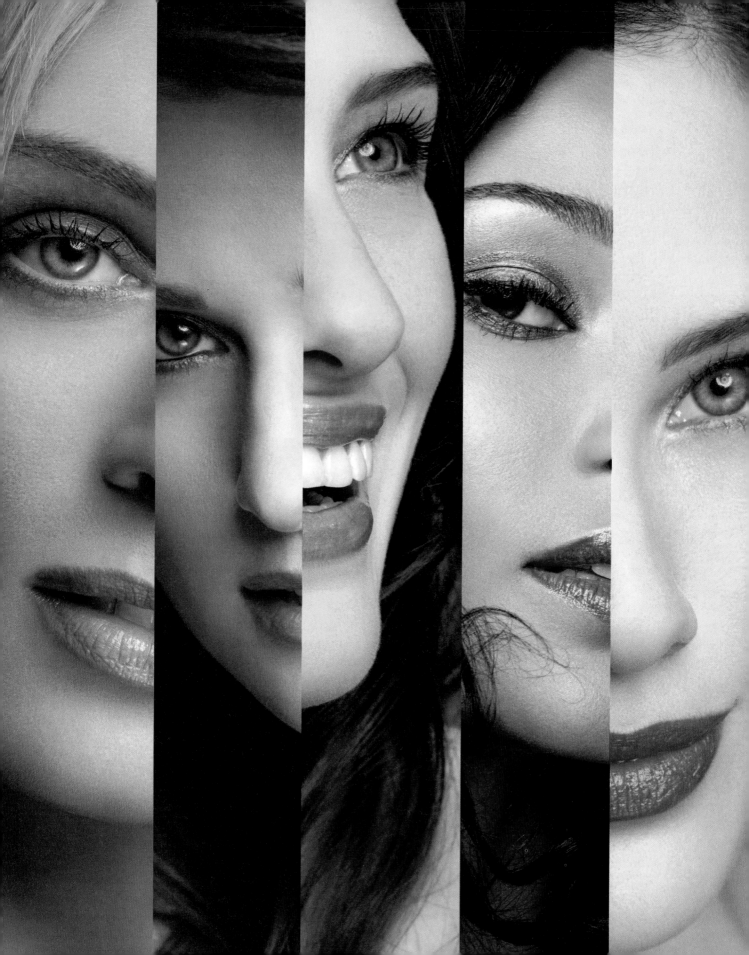

A good woman is a wondrous creature, cleaving to
the right and to the good under all change.
—ALFRED, LORD TENNYSON

chapter twelve makeup your mood

Too often women get a bum rap for being moody. Upbeat, serious, silly, sad, sexy, stubborn, gung ho-and that's just me on any given day! I wouldn't be me without my varied moods, and you wouldn't be you without yours. All hail moodiness!

We need to think of our diverse emotions as a positive aspect of our feminine nature. After all, our shifting experiences and feelings are what give texture and excitement to our lives. Rather than dismiss them, let's embrace our moods and enhance our looks accordingly! By varying how we use makeup, we can better express our feelings, set free our fantasies, and show the world what multifaceted, fascinating creatures we are.

With our increasing responsibilities, women today don't have enough opportunities to just be playful. Makeup is an accessible, safe vehicle for exploration and a powerful channel for self-expression. So let's bring back that free-spirited way we used to think about makeup when we were young and experiment avidly with products and looks.

By being playful with cosmetics, we not only change our appearance, we shift how others perceive us. I say keep 'em guessing! Plus, switching up your makeup can help support taking a different approach to a challenging day or night. Are we talking empowerment through eyeliner? You bet.

Now that you've mastered your feature focus techniques, it's time to expand your makeup repertoire to create special looks that match whatever "beauty mood" you're in. Let's play!

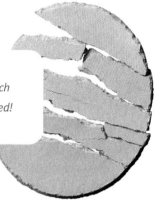

Beauty Mood: Romantic

Fairy tales can come true—especially when you play the heroine and look the part. A soft Renaissance face with rosy lips and cheeks and soft eyes conjures up visions of love and romance. Think ethereal Botticelli beauty. Ah, lovely! And a great choice for cheeks-focused maidens.

Start off by applying primer, foundation, under-eye concealer, blemish concealer (if needed), and powder. Next, sweep a light pink highlighter powder under the eyebrow and on the inner corners of the eyes. Sweep the same highlighter on top of the cheekbones.

Keep eyes soft and doelike by sweeping on a neutral brown shade across the lid and smudging a little under the lower lash line. Skip the eyeliner, as it's too harsh for this sweet look. Finish with black mascara on the top and bottom lashes.

Next, rosy up the apples of your cheeks with a healthy application of flowery rose powder blush. Swirl it on in circular motions for that shy, winsomely blushing look.

Create lips a man would die to kiss by dabbing on a moisturizing lipstick in the same rosy shade as your blush, using your fingertip for the lightest touch. With a pretty pout like that, prepare to be swept off your feet in a swirl of smooches!

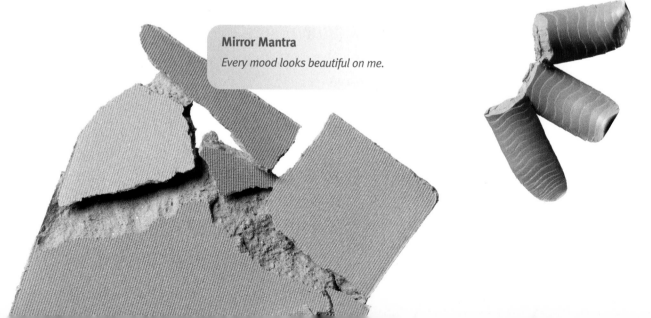

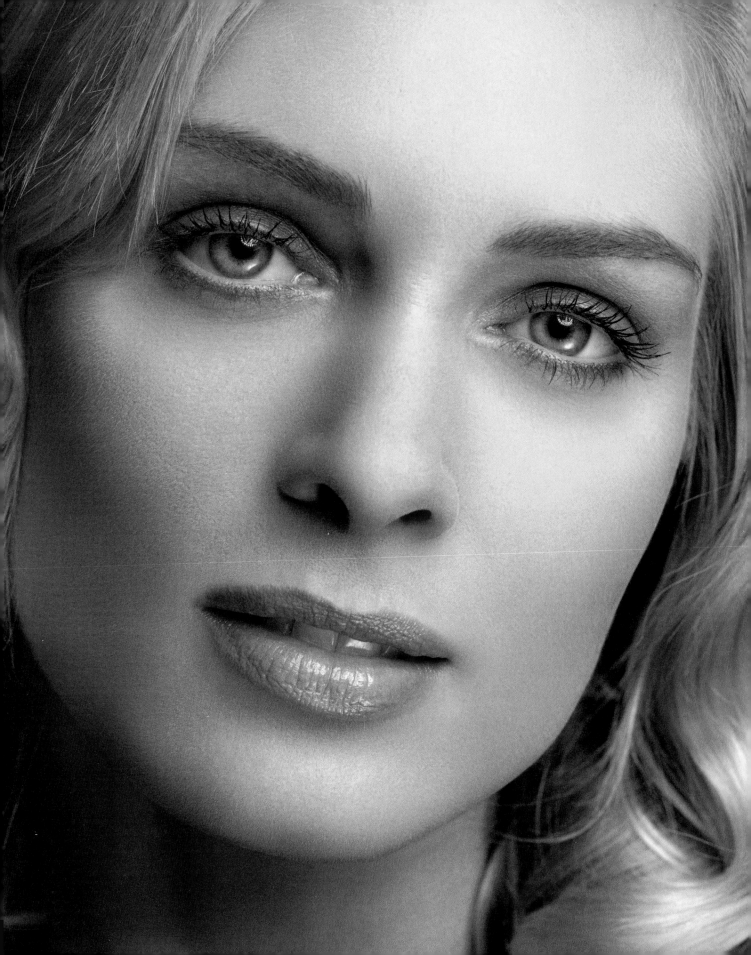

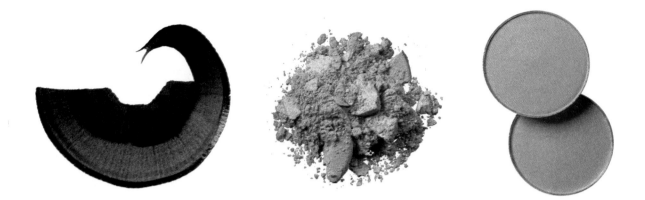

Beauty Mood: Seductive

You start noticing the signs well before nightfall. Your walk becomes a spellbinding sway. Your skin takes note of every breeze and rustle of fabric. Oh, hot mama, you're feeling extra sexy. Positively intoxicating. And combustible!

When you're smokin', a smoldering gaze only adds fuel to your fire. Rim those eyes with kohl, and any man is at your mercy. Just promise to use your powers for good, you vixen!

Achieving a captivating look is not nearly as complicated as mastering the art of seduction. Follow these eyes-focused steps (and your heart), and success will be yours.

Start with primer, foundation, and blemish concealer (if needed). Leave the under-eye concealer for later. Apply powder everywhere except right under the eyes. You'll see why in a minute.

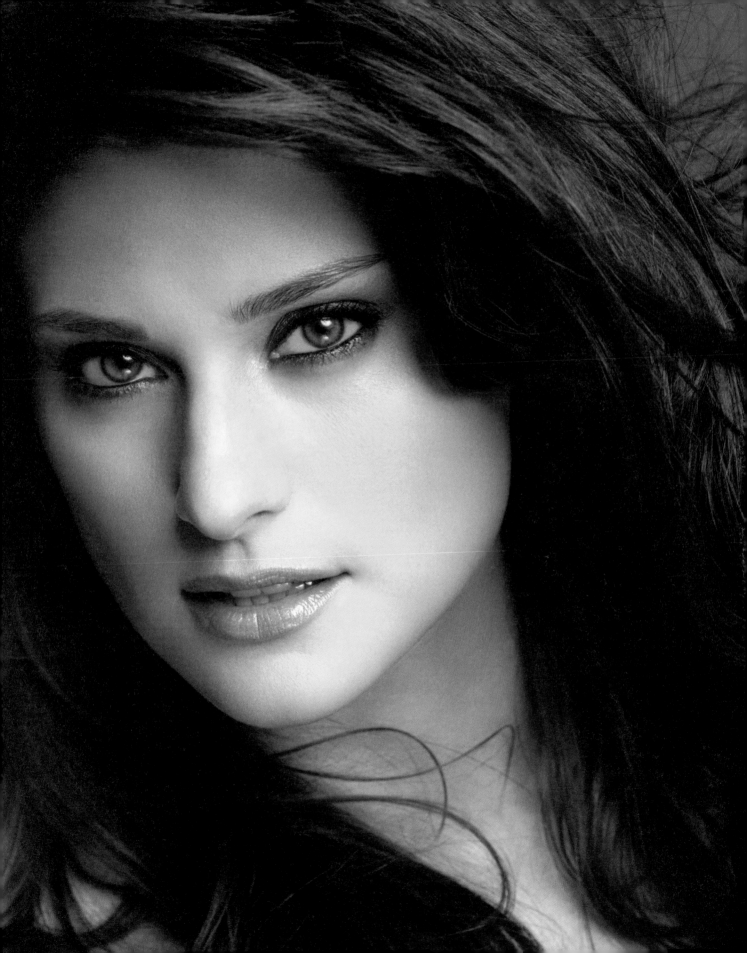

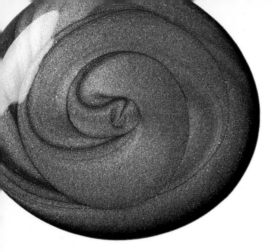

Next, begin smudging dark eyeliner on the upper lash line as close to the roots as possible and on the inside rim of the eyes.

Now sweep on a dark contour shade of eye shadow across the lid from the lash line to the crease, and use an angle brush to apply the same shade under the lower lash line. Blend on a midtone eye shadow across the crease. Place a highlight shade under the brow and on the inner corners of the eyes. The gradation of color from darkest at the lashes to lightest under the brow is what gives this look its intensity.

Apply black mascara on the top and the bottom lashes. Smooth away any traces of shadow that may have fallen beneath the eyes with a nonlatex sponge dipped into a bit of under-eye concealer (my magic eraser trick). Then sweep the lightest application of powder under the eyes to set it.

Keep the rest of your makeup simple so the eyes steal the seductive show. Lightly sweep on a powder blush in a soft color, and apply a nude or neutral shade of lip gloss. Ravishing.

Now swing those hips out the door, you passionate minx!

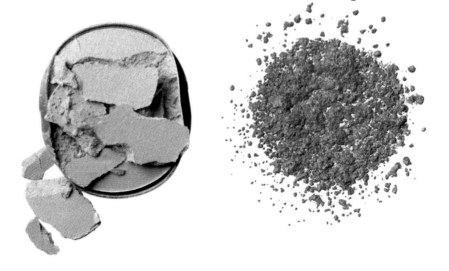

Carmindy Fan Q&A

Q: *My green eyes are large, and I also have highly arched eyebrows. How can I achieve a smoky-eye look without it looking like a black eye? I usually only wear neutral makeup.*

—Barbara, 39, Kennett Square, PA

A: You don't always need to use black or charcoal shades to create a smoky eye. Go for a subtler version by using shades of purple to accentuate your green eyes. Line the eyes with a dark amethyst pencil and then apply a dark shadow in the same color family across the lid. Now blend on a midtone shadow across the crease; this will soften the color on the lid slightly. Sweep a highlight shade under the brow and on the inside corners, then finish with black mascara. Devastating!

Q: *I always like dark, dramatic eyes, but I have trouble evening out under my eyes with concealer. I can still see some gray. What to do?*

—Lucy, 23, San Francisco, CA

A: A great trick is to apply foundation on your eyelids and under your eyes. Then apply powder only to the lids. Next, sweep on your liner, eye shadows, and mascara. After your eye makeup is complete, apply under-eye concealer, and set it with powder. This method allows you to sweep away any bits of eye shadow that may have fallen during application and even out any natural darkness in one go.

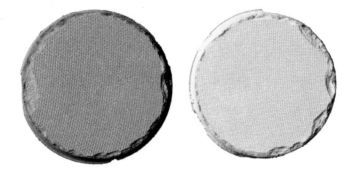

Beauty Mood: Strong and Take Charge

Oh, girl, get your red on.

Ever hear about power dressing? This is a face fit for conquering and victory dancing. Whether you're headed to a big meeting or a meet-up with an intriguing suitor, working a red lipstick communicates strength and take-charge confidence. Call it the red-alert factor: people pay attention to words spoken from fearless, scarlet lips. Make yours positively memorable.

Start by following the basic steps: apply primer, foundation, blemish/under-eye concealer (if needed), and powder.

Keep eye makeup minimal so your mouth remains the focal point. Sweep a vanilla-colored eye shadow across the entire lid, and trace the upper lash line with a chocolate-colored eyeliner. A light smudge of taupe shadow in the crease and under the lower lash line is all you need for definition. Follow with black mascara on the top lashes only.

For cheeks, apply a very subtle, natural-looking blush. If you use cream blush, apply it before your face powder.

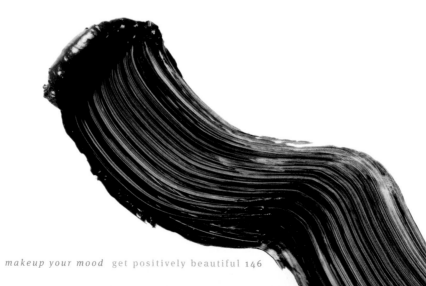

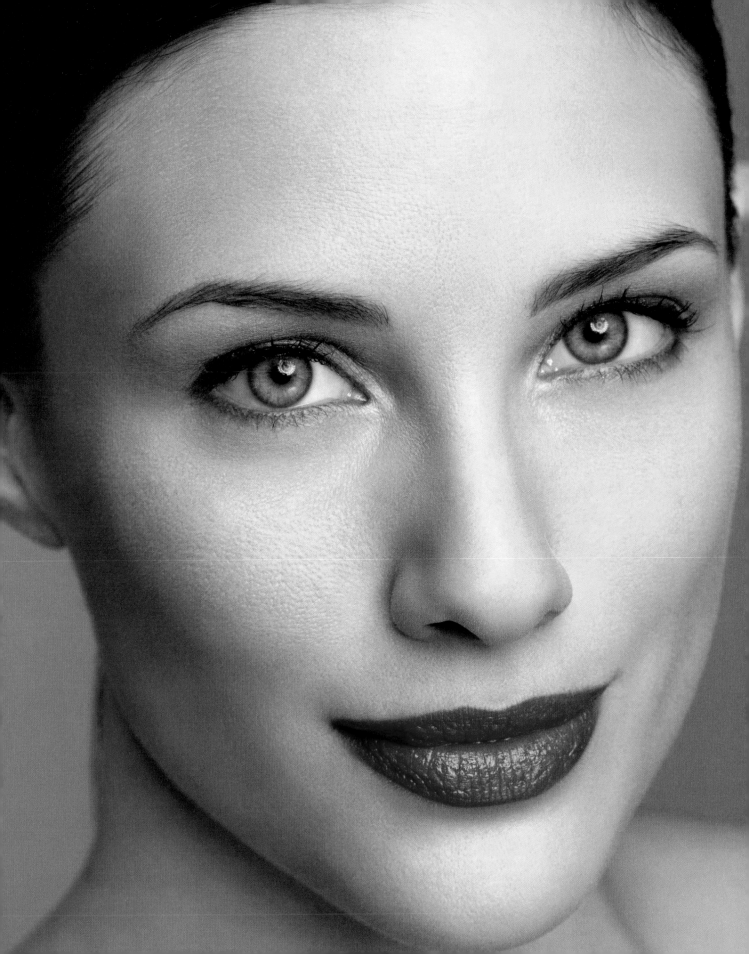

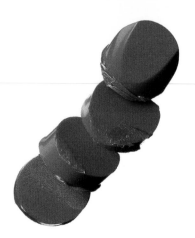

Next, choose a red lipstick that complements your skin tone. Think blue-based reds for fair-skinned women, true reds for olive-skinned women, and deeper blood reds for dark-skinned women. If you're a redhead with a fair but warm complexion, head for brick or tomato reds.

Prepare a long-lasting power pucker by first tracing the lip line with a nude or clear lip pencil. This keeps lipstick in place and helps avoid color bleeding.

Next, paint your lips red with precision by using a lip brush. Blot carefully and reapply for a glistening, velvet finish. (I never add gloss over red lipstick; it's too overwhelming. Let the color alone do the talking here.) If you're looking to command the room but want to take a more subtle approach, go for a red lip tint or a sheer red lipstick.

Classic, classy, and oh so sassy—that's you, my ruby beauty!

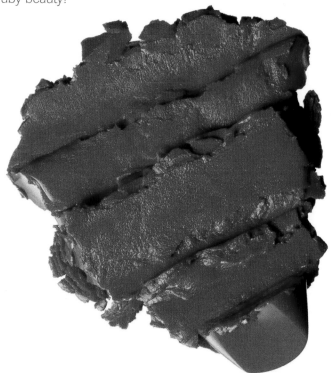

Carmindy Fan Q&A

Q: *I have a medium complexion and full Latina lips. Which red lipstick won't make me look like a clown? Most of the ones I've tried make me feel like Bozo, and I end up wearing nude or light shades most of the time.*

—Wendy, 34, Puerto Rico

A: When you're feeling like you want to show off those full, fabulous lips, try a deep *sheer* red. The sheer factor allows your skin to show through, so you gain the color punch without feeling like you're auditioning for Ringling Brothers.

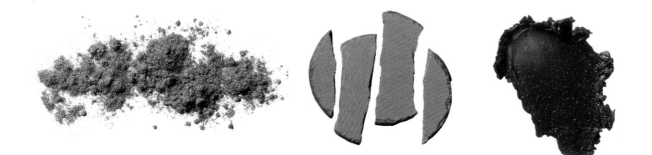

Beauty Mood: Fabulous

When you're feeling absolutely unstoppable, accelerate your fabulousity by going full-on glam! This is no time for dainty, my lady. Indulge your need for the hot and the new with a trendy trick or two. Playing with liquid eyeliner shows that you're on the cutting edge of fashion and about to reach the stratosphere of stupendous!

Start with your canvas basics: primer, foundation, blemish and under-eye concealer (if needed), and powder.

Now for the fun part: liquid eyeliner. Try exciting shades that work well for day or night, like teal, eggplant, sapphire blue, or teak brown. Classic black is always great for a fabulous evening statement.

Starting at the inner corners of the eyes, sweep liner across the upper lash line and end with a little wing at the outer corners. (By applying the eyeliner first, you can correct any smudges without redoing your whole eye look. Go slowly, and you'll be gorgeous in no time.)

After the liner is completely dry, apply a sparkling midtone eye shadow across the lid from the lash line to the crease, and smudge the same color under the lower lash line. Smooth on highlighter under the brow, and apply black mascara on the top and bottom lashes for a flirty fringe.

Cheeks can be brought to their full potential with neutral blush swept across the cheekbones and highlighter swept on top of the cheekbones.

Finish with a dazzling lip-gloss-of-the-moment and—voila—you are *utterly* chic!

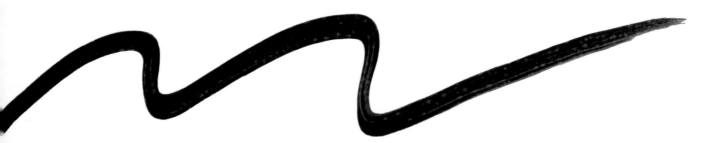

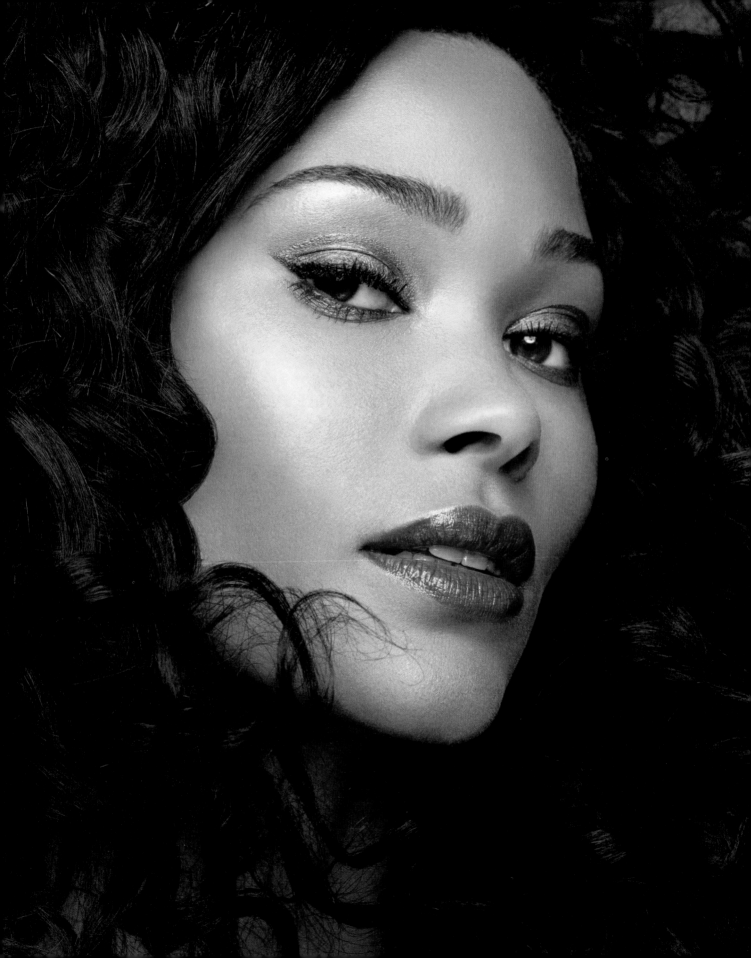

Beauty Mood: Carefree

Blessed are the days when we awaken with that happy-go-lucky feeling where nothing, but nothing, can bring us down. As a tried-and-true beach girl, such times bring back memories of twirling down a sandy beach with waves lapping at my feet. Bliss!

A bronzy, golden look is the face to match this magically in-tune mood. Best of all, a kissed-by-the-sun, back-from-vacation glow can be yours at any time. Just skip along through these steps, my mellowed-out honey.

Start with the basics: primer, foundation, blemish and under-eye concealer (if needed), and powder.

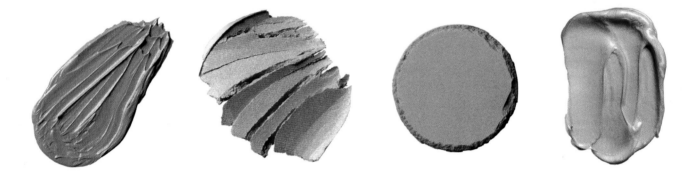

Now blend on a bronzer (before powder, if it's a cream bronzer) to the temples, along the sides of the face, and under the hollows of the cheeks. Blend a tad across the bridge of your nose for an extra touch of sunshine.

Next, apply a light gold highlighter on top of the cheekbones and across the entire eyelid, from the lash line to under the brow bone, and on the inner corners of the eyes.

Apply bronzy brown eyeliner across the upper lash line, and smudge a bit under the lower lash line as well. Finish off with black mascara on the top lashes only.

Swirl on a coral blush to the apples of the cheeks and sweep on a peachy tinted lip balm for a super-carefree mood or a coral sheer lip gloss if you care a little more.

Now throw up your arms and shout with glee, *I'm me, I'm free, oh blessed be!* Cartwheels optional but encouraged!

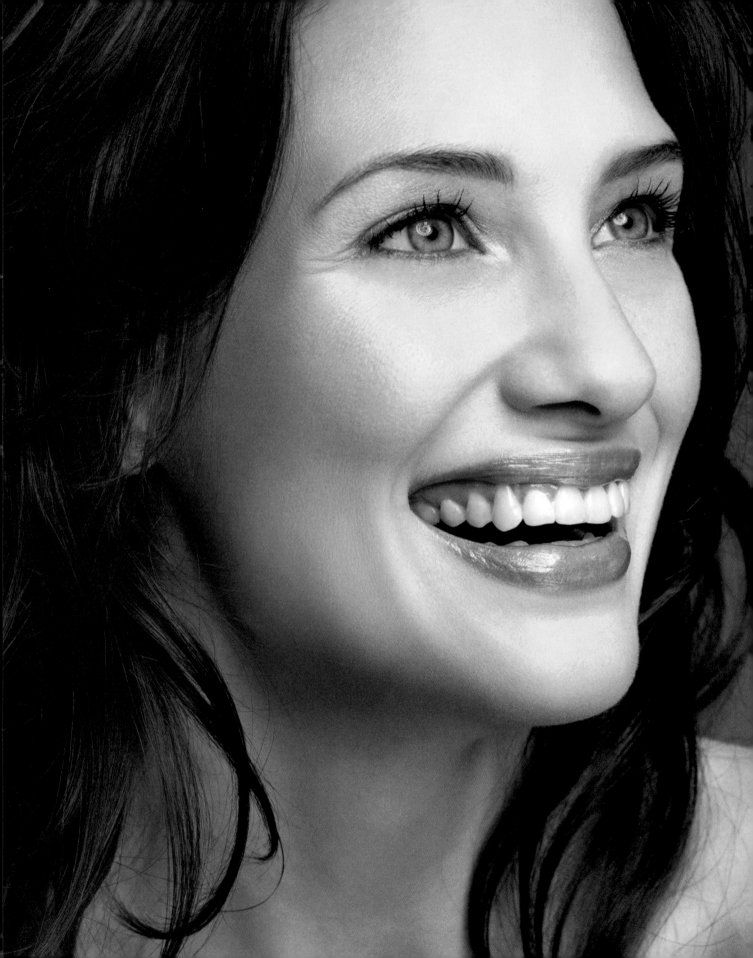

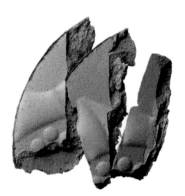

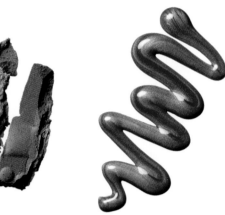

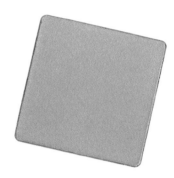

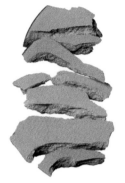

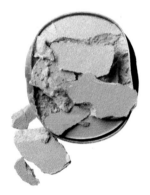

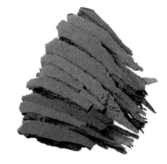

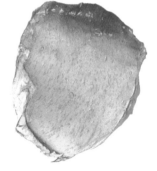

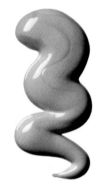

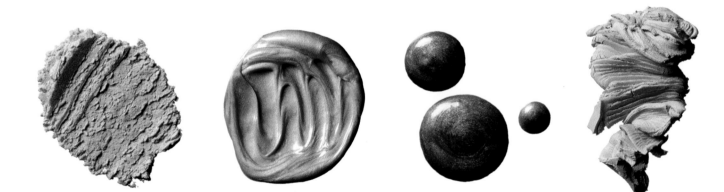

chapter thirteen
everyone loves a makeover

Oh, the energy of true beauty! That's what these ladies offer.

Some have been friends of mine for years; some I just met. All of them are at different stages in their lives, yet each one is a powerhouse in her own right.

I love women like these—women like you!

Sarah, 28

HOMETOWN: SALT LAKE CITY, UTAH

When I was in first grade, I developed alopecia and my eyelashes fell out. By the time I became a teenager, I felt like a freak. I overcompensated by obsessively grooming my eyebrows—they were in my control. On my wedding day, the makeup artist said, "Hey, it's no big deal. Just wear eyeliner." So I did and still do every day. When I look at the pictures now, I forget the lashes; I just see the joy.

Beauty magazines used to influence me, especially the stories about the "ideal" oval face shape; mine is round and I hated it! I remember thinking if I could suck in my cheeks at night and sleep like that, my chipmunk cheeks would disappear. I considered contouring my face to make it look more slender. But I don't have the patience to do that every day. And why should I?

I feel okay about my face, but am still working on loving it.

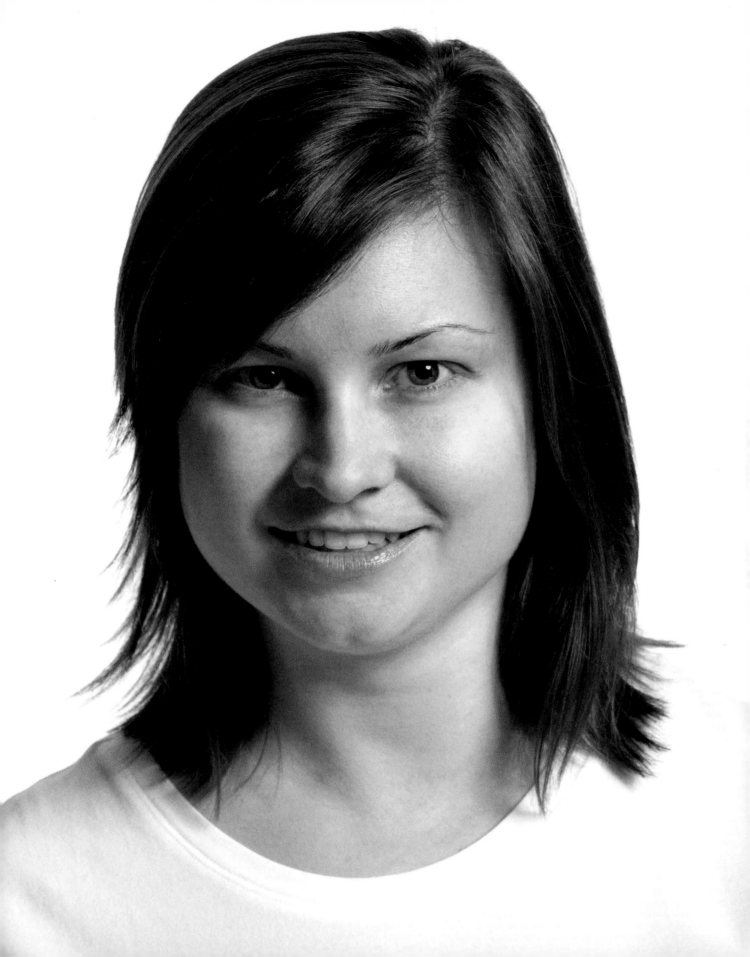

Carmindy Vision: What I See

Sarah's cheeks are my favorites! When she smiles, her face lights up—drawing my eye to her flawless, smooth skin. And you know, I didn't notice Sarah's sparse lashes until she pointed them out.

I wanted to play up her eyes and cheekbones to accentuate the upper half of her face—spotlighting her natural beauty and turning up her confidence.

Instead of trying to re-create or change Sarah by gluing on false lashes, I smudged a shadow on her lash line for a soft, lovely take on definition. It's a simple technique she can easily repeat at home.

Sarah overplucked her brows. No worries. A bit of brow corrector brought them back to an elegant shape—framing her eyes perfectly.

For those gorgeous cheeks, I placed shimmering highlight on the cheekbones, then swept powder bronzer along the temples and under the cheekbones. The finishing pop of floral blush on the apples gave Sarah a sweet and stunning look.

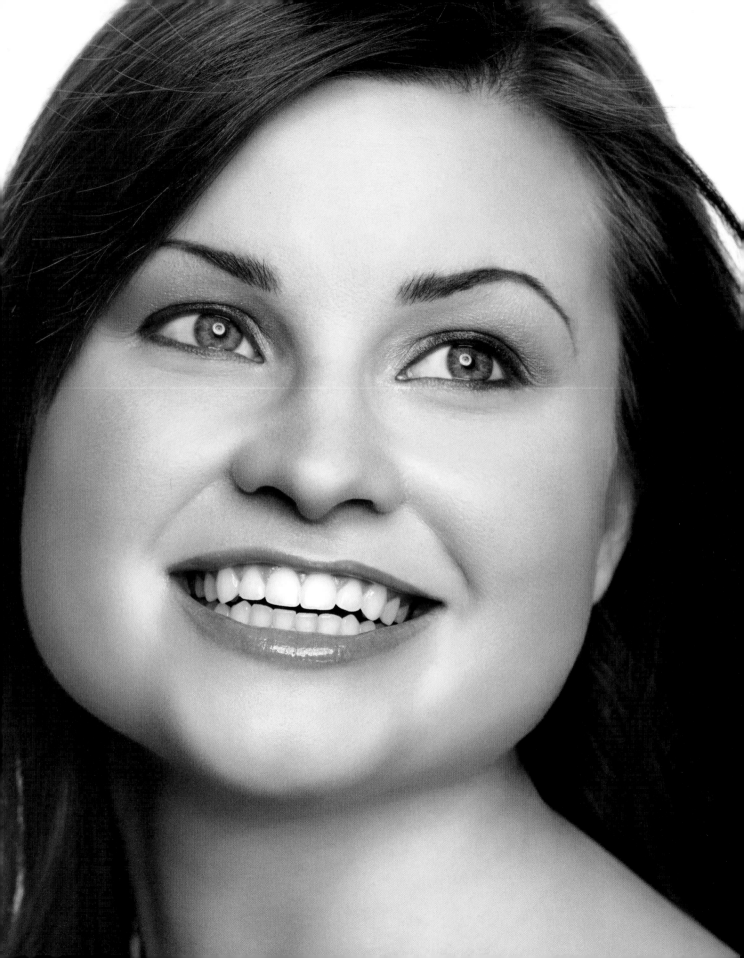

Khrystine, 33

My fiancé and I just returned from a fourteen-month journey around the world. The experience transformed my approach to beauty. I used to be super high maintenance about grooming—Ms. Mani-Pedi USA. I read all the fashion magazines and spent untold sums on expensive makeup.

But during our adventure, we were so involved in meeting people, going scuba diving, and exploring cultures, I let most of my regimen go. I was radiating beauty because I was doing so many beautiful things.

Today I define a beautiful woman as one who's kind, very natural, and confident in her own worth. When a woman carries herself with gentle strength, she's stunning.

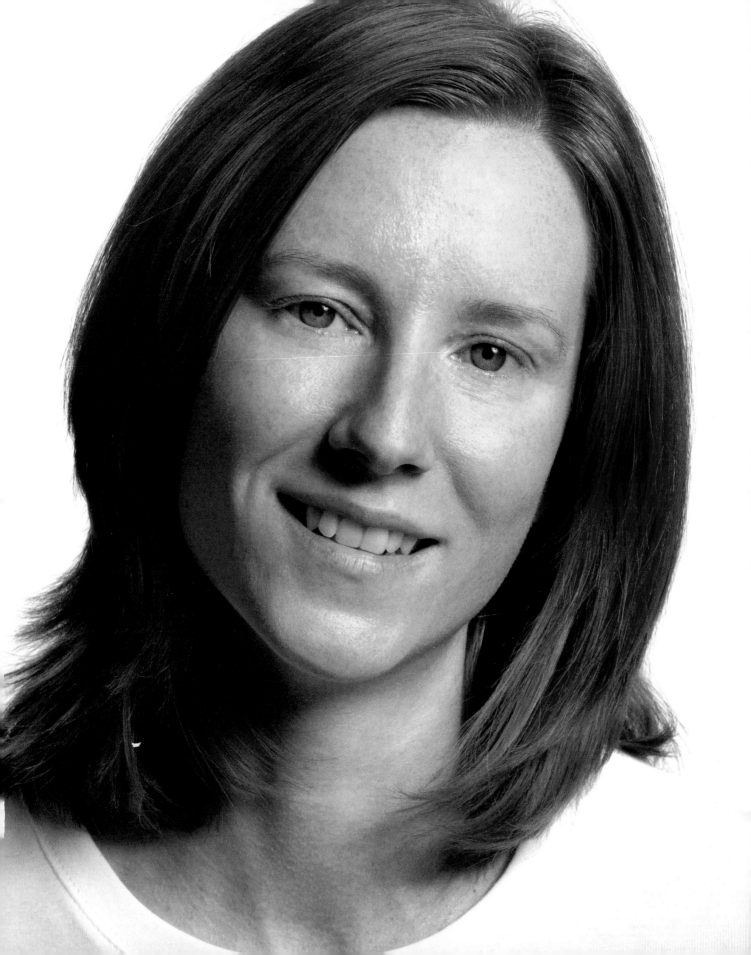

Carmindy Vision: What I See

Khrystine reminds me of summertime. Beautiful skin with youthful freckles, amazing eyes, and what coloring!

Khrystine exudes natural sophistication. I chose a 5-minute face for her because she's a busy business-woman as well as a world traveler. She needs to be able to jet off at a moment's notice looking fresh, not fussy.

I smoothed on liquid foundation and set it with a dusting of powder. Next, I placed highlight under her brows, on the inside corners of her eyes, and on her cheekbones. I smudged chocolate brown pencil (the perfect contrast for her baby blues) along the upper lash line and a bit under the lower lash line. A healthy dose of mascara showed how her blonde lashes were really a mile long.

Playing into her warm coloring, a pop of peachy pink blush on the apples of her cheeks revealed how "wow" her cheekbones are. And a peachy pink lip gloss set off her inviting smile. Polished, pretty perfection!

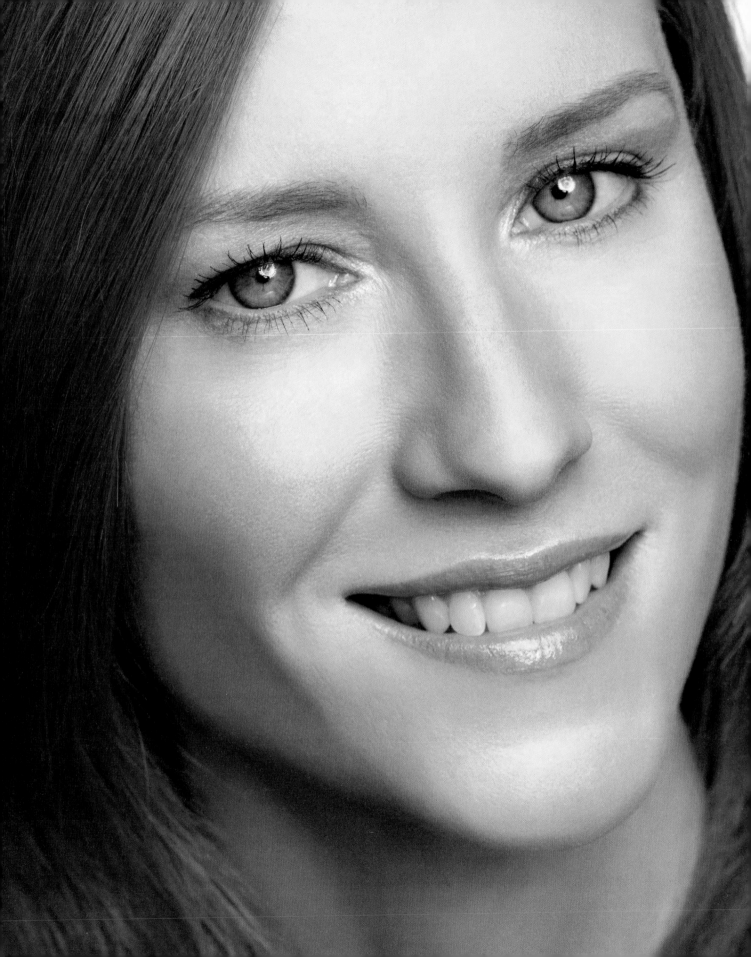

Katherine, 50

HOMETOWN: LOS ANGELES, CALIFORNIA

When I was a child, total strangers would come up to my mother and say, "Oh, what a pretty little girl." I remember that happening once when I was about eight. After accepting the compliment, my mother walked me down the street and said in no uncertain terms, "Just because you're pretty doesn't mean you'll get everything." From that moment on, I connected beauty with shame. Beauty wasn't to be trusted, let alone counted on. I disassociated from my looks for the next forty-one years.

I believed my spirit was beautiful, but not my face, so I didn't even attempt to play into my assets. Instead, I played the "jolly girl" role in my younger years. Even into my thirties and forties, men would hit on me, saying I was breathtaking, and I still didn't believe it.

It's only been in the past year or so that I've clicked back into my beauty. Now I own my features and love wearing makeup. If I could be reincarnated, I would want to come back with the same face. I'm gorgeous!

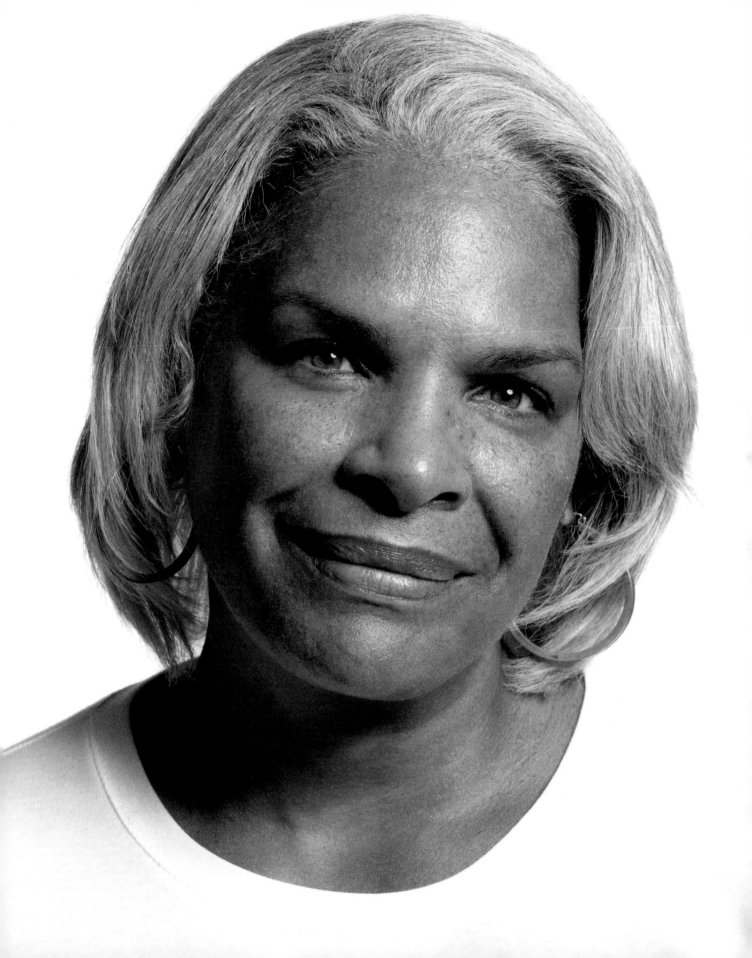

Carmindy Vision: What I See

My goodness, what power words have over our self-image. To learn that my dear friend Kathy spent so many years feeling ashamed of her beauty is unbelievable. A crime!

From the moment I met her, I was fascinated by Kathy's face. Her skin is glorious, and those eyes and cheekbones create such drama. She can wear any look with ease; a true playhouse for a makeup artist like me.

On her eyes, I used a shimmering pale gold shadow as highlight, smoothed on a copper shade that works with her skin tone, and put liquid liner on her upper lash line for drama. Women over thirty can play with shimmer as long as it's pearlescent because it won't settle into fine lines and will instead bring light to the face. A raisin blush accentuated her amazing cheekbones. And for a soft lip, just a touch of gloss in a sunset shade.

It's so wonderful to see Kathy now embracing the power of her own beauty.

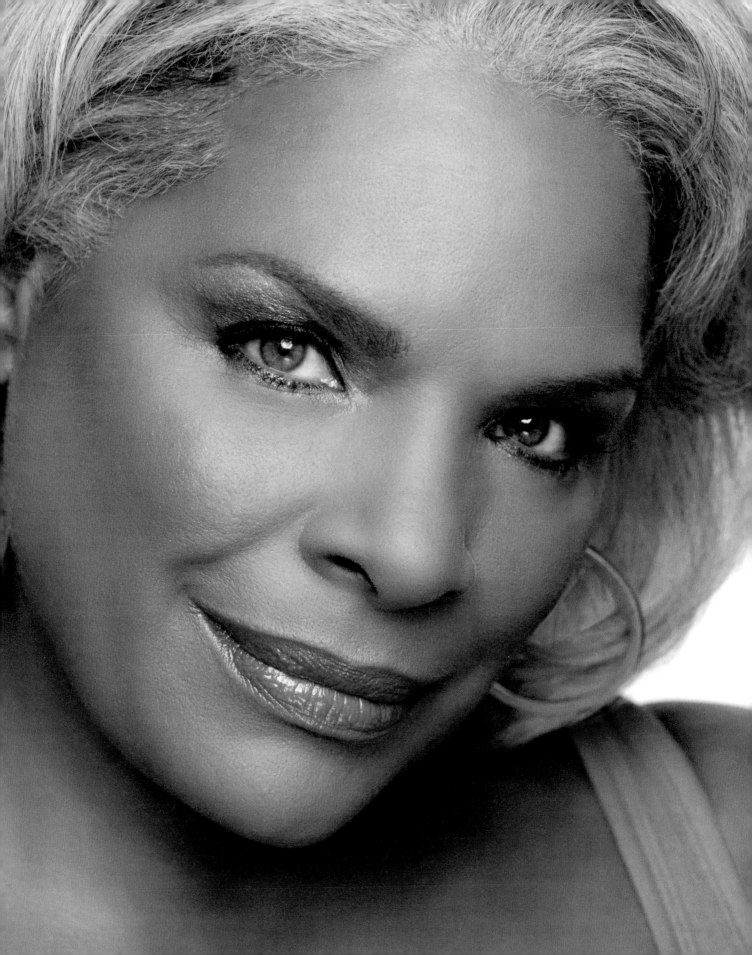

Michelle, 36

HOMETOWN: PACIFIC PALISADES, CALIFORNIA

In hindsight, I credit my mom for my strong self-image. She always told me I was pretty, but she also emphasized that beauty comes from the inside out. Growing up, though, I took her words with a grain of salt. I mean, don't all moms think their daughters are lovely?

In my twenties, I entered the fashion industry and spent my days photographing models. While I understood the illusion and handiwork that goes into a shoot, I still found myself looking in the mirror and feeling inadequate by comparison. Luckily I didn't let it break my stride as a sexy, confident woman.

Nowadays I worry a little about the aging process. But when I consider all the treatments and drama, I stop and remember how blessed I am with role models. My grandmother—who's in her eighties—is amazingly beautiful and very assured. I hold fast to that!

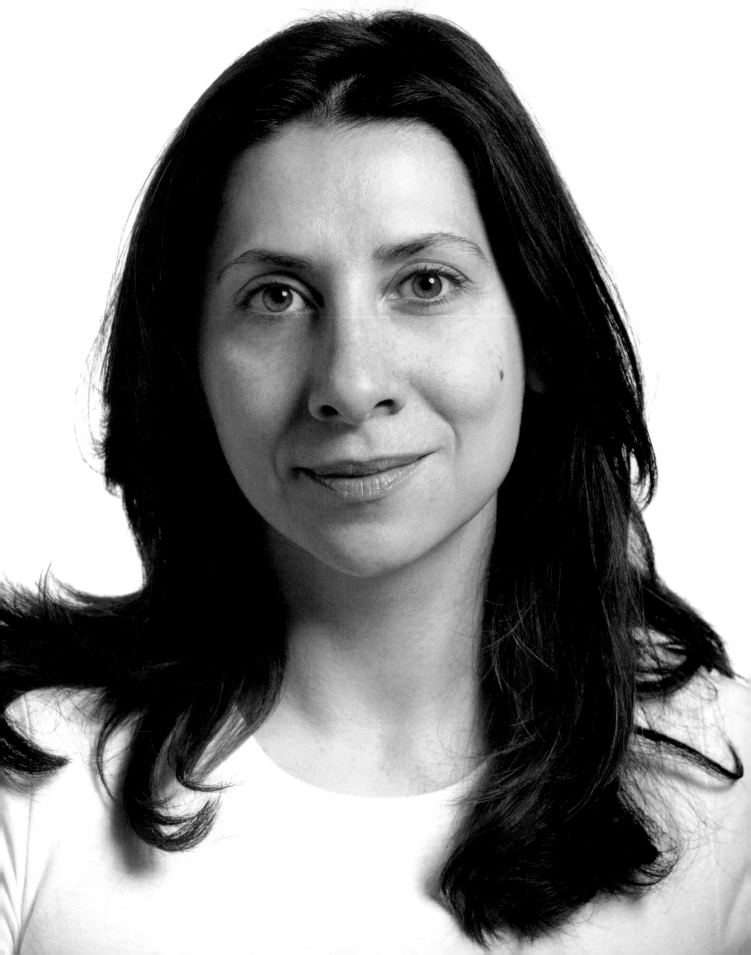

Carmindy Vision: What I See

As my best friend, Michelle has always inspired me with her unfailing confidence, natural sex appeal, and ability to love herself. She explodes with energy and passion for life. She's unstoppable!

Michelle is a lashes enthusiast. So we decided to go all out for an incredibly sexy, of-the-moment eye look that's sixties retro with a modern twist. I layered liquid liner on her upper lash line, applied a few false eyelashes at the corners, and followed with a triple coat of black mascara to really play up her best feature.

We balanced her look with soft cheek and lip colors to keep those lashes the stars of the Michelle Show. Absolutely fabulous!

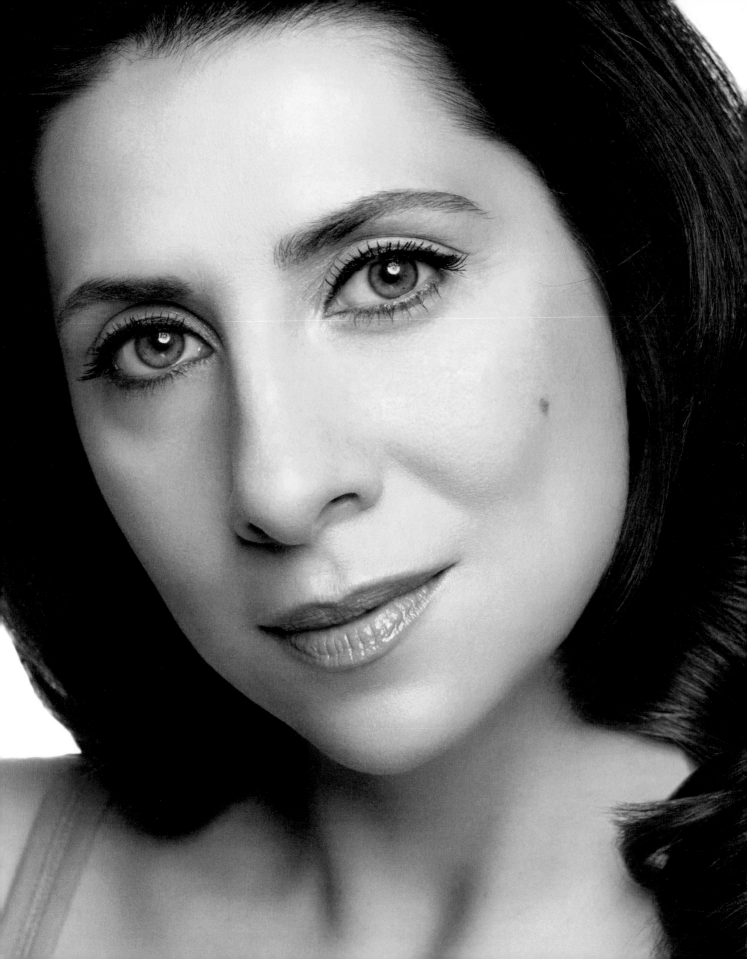

Ivonne, 52

HOMETOWN: MIAMI, FLORIDA

Growing up in the Cuban community, I felt very unappealing because I was a skinny, gawky kid. I developed a distorted self-image. Conversely, I didn't have typical Latina coloring, with my light eyes and hair, yet received compliments on that.

I read *Vogue* and *Harper's Bazaar.* I lived for them. My mother also hugely influenced me. She had an eye and worked her own style so well. Very Jackie O with gloves and a hat and a shift. Terribly chic! I paid attention—and still do—to clothes, much more so than to any beauty regimen per se.

Today people compliment me on my skin, and I feel very good about that. In fact, I think this is the best I've ever looked. It has to do with being this age. It's the most powerful time for women. We can become exactly who we are rather than having to please anyone else or fit with any particular role. Change can be frightening, but it is so liberating.

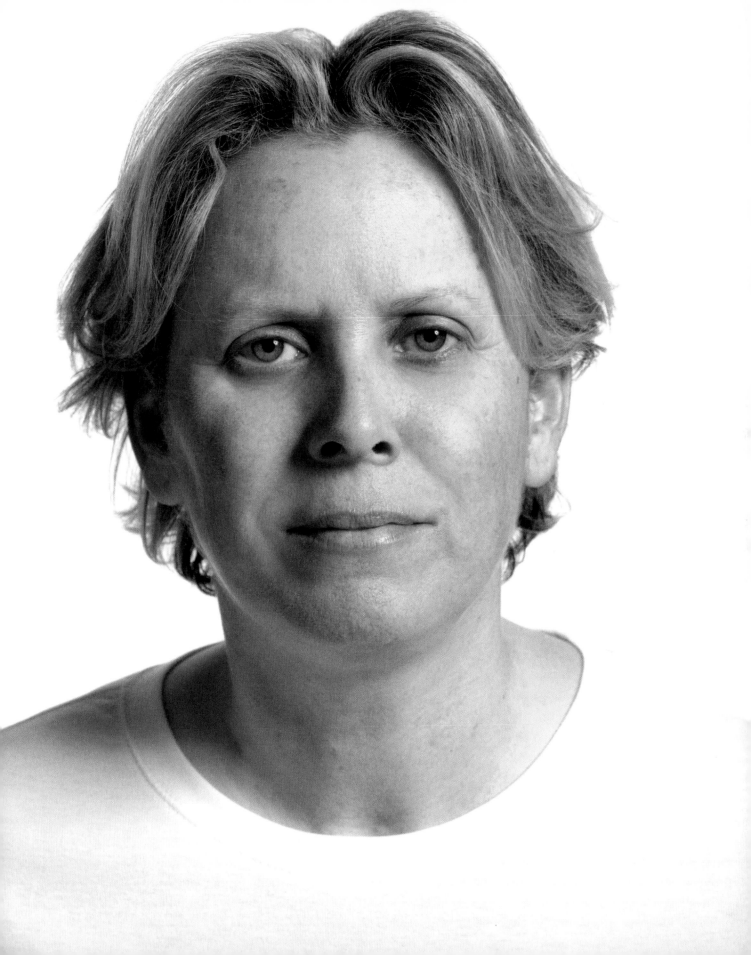

Carmindy Vision: What I See

When I met Ivonne, I fell in love with her eyes and skin. She has such a balanced face, with perfect almond-shaped eyes and symmetrical features. She's a strong woman who radiates beauty.

Like many women her age, Ivonne's hormones are in flux, and she experiences hot flashes several times each day. By starting with a luminizing face primer, her foundation will stay fresh, and any extra shine will be kept under control throughout the day.

As a Latina with light coloring, Ivonne's blonde lashes and brows tend to wash her out. I deepened her brow color and lined her upper lash line to showcase the shape of her eyes and give them a wide-awake vitality.

A soft quartz eye shadow brought out her lovely blue-green eyes without being overpowering. A pink-tinted lip balm played into her natural lip color; it's a low-maintenance way to keep her lips supple and colorful all day. Smart and sassy!

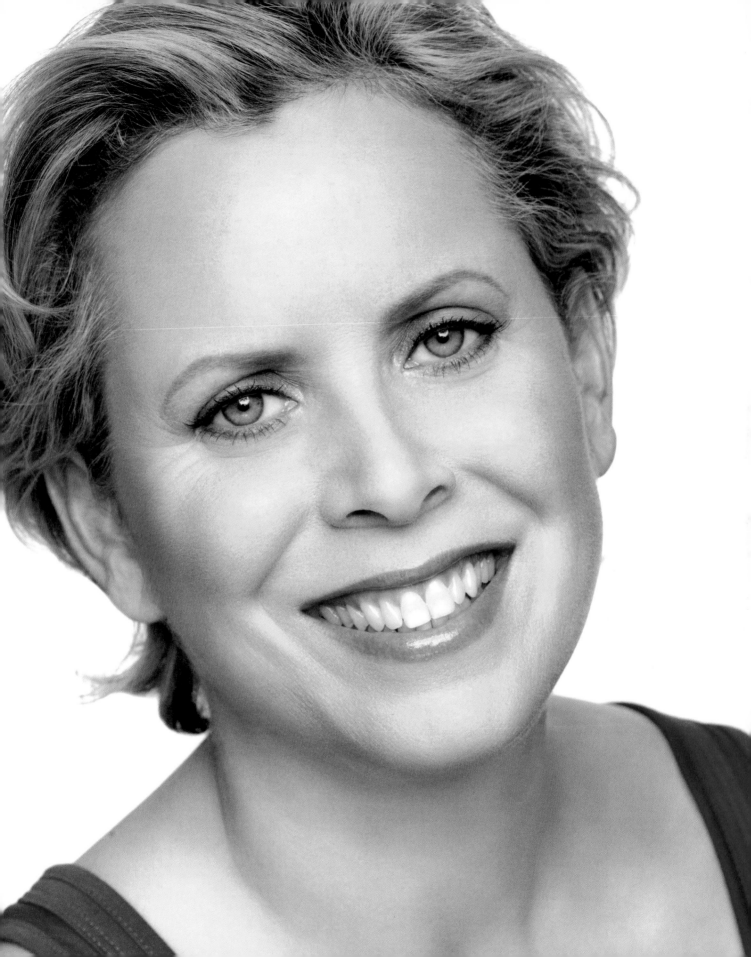

Joy, 39

HOMETOWN: DES MOINES, IOWA

Looks weren't commented on in my family, good or bad. Academic performance mattered; a strong work ethic was what counted. So I didn't grow up with a poor perception of my appearance, but I didn't understand the power of beauty either.

I only started appreciating my face once I reached my thirties. I have unusual features: a prominent nose, an expansive forehead, brows with a mind of their own. Rather than try to alter or cover up these traits, I've made them my signature. Who wants to look like a celebrity clone?

I may be late to the makeup party, but I really enjoy playing with different looks. It's fun to be a femme fatale one day, a doe-eyed innocent the next. I'm also a fanatic about skin care and go to a threading salon to keep the brows groomed, but never tamed! Now I pay attention when I see another woman with a cockeyed brow. I think, "Oh look, another member of the tribe; I bet *she's* an interesting lady . . ."

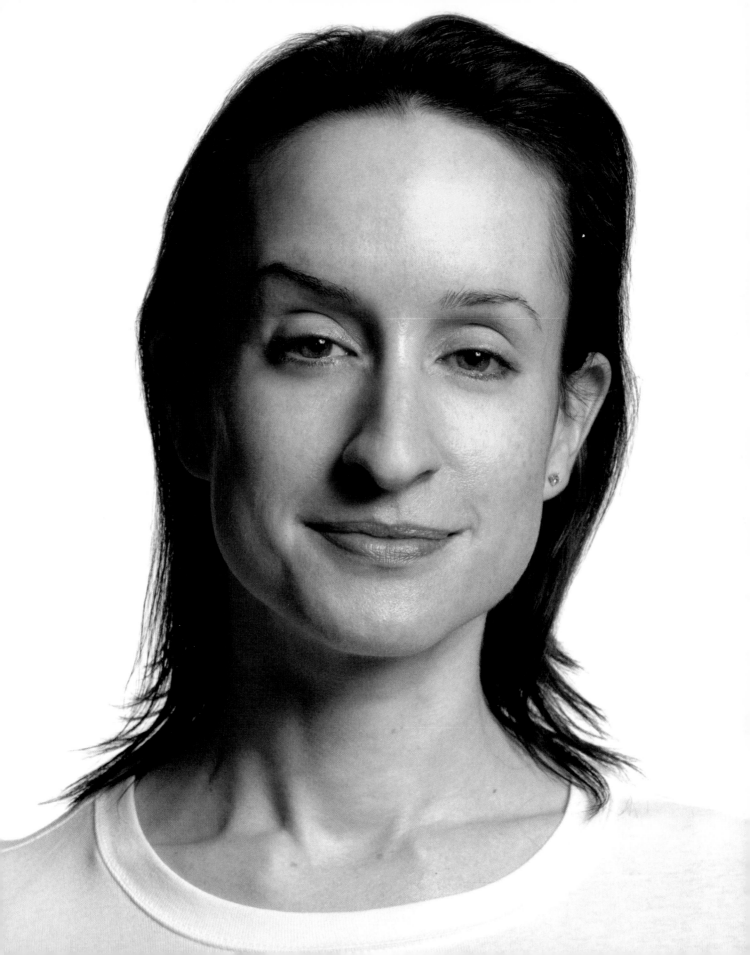

Carmindy Vision: What I See

Joy has a face that is so emotionally transparent. If she's feeling it, her face shows it with honesty. Those eyebrows express her intelligence and passion. She has such a regal, beautiful look. Breathtaking.

Inspired by Joy's dramatic brow and hazel eyes, I decided to create a modern smoky eye. The new approach is to use autumn shadow shades in khaki, green, and gold instead of the traditional black and gray palette. When paired with black liquid liner and mascara, these colors create a smoldering, more sophisticated effect.

I finished with a bit of orchid blush and sheer mauve lip gloss for pure sex appeal. Shazam, ma'am. Joy's inner diva exploded on camera. I think we unleashed a vixen!

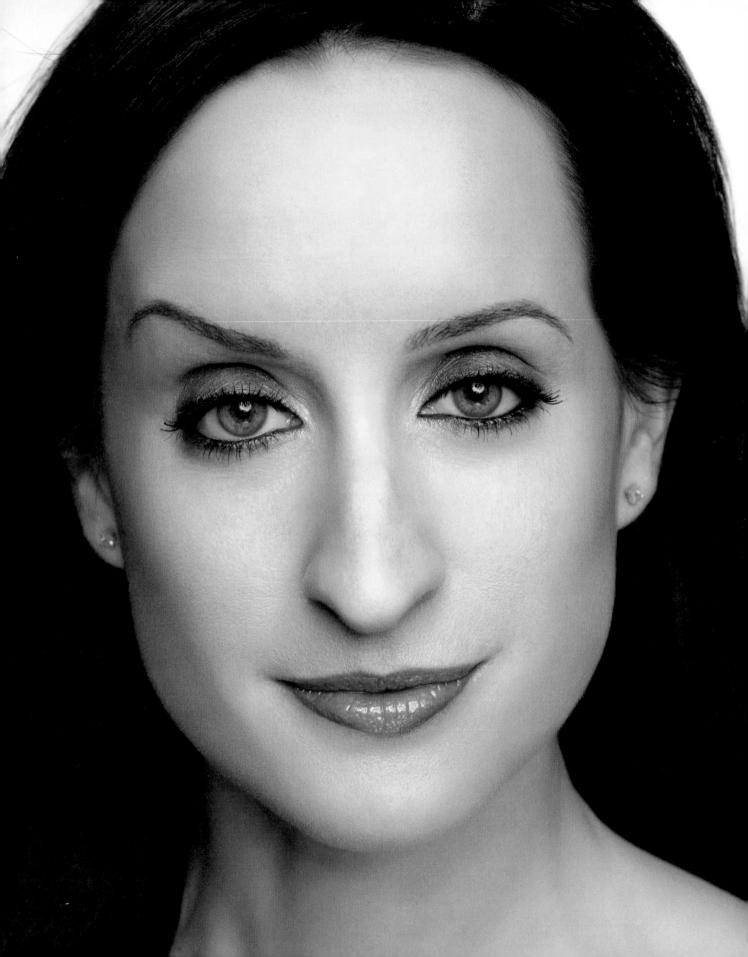

Lois, 68

HOMETOWN: MOUNT VERNON, NEW YORK

I grew up with a stunningly beautiful mother. Throughout my youth, people would comment on how I was pretty, but not as pretty as her. They'd say, "Oh, you have such nice blue eyes, but not as blue as your mother's." After a while, I just withdrew from the whole beauty game; I didn't want to compete.

Once I reached my thirties, I stopped making excuses about who I was and started to own my face. Nowadays I feel like an oddball among my friends because I haven't had cosmetic surgery. Even though I'm not thrilled with all of the changes that aging brings, I still want to look like me. I want a face that can still be expressive and smile freely!

For me, feeling beautiful means feeling healthy, having confidence in myself, and being in touch with my spirituality. That's what truly counts.

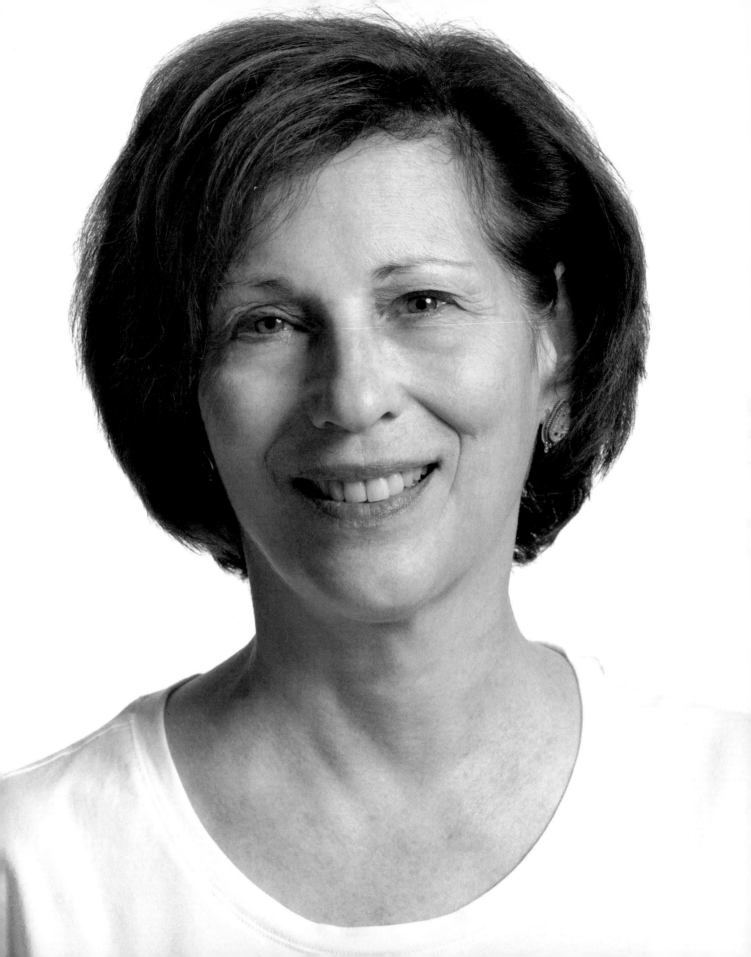

Carmindy Vision: What I See

Lois is amazing. The epitome of a whole woman. Her face speaks to what she's accomplished and the wisdom that's come along the way. I applaud her resistance to surgery. Who wants to look in the mirror and say, "I don't know who that person is"?

Lois's eyes are captivating and whoa, what outrageous bone structure. I wanted to highlight her elegance by playing up those cheekbones and baby blues.

First, luminizing face primer bounced light around her complexion, softening her fine lines. Lois has such great skin, I applied only the sheerest veil of foundation.

A touch of cream blush on the apples of her cheeks brought the radiance back to the dry areas common in most mature women. I used a nude lip liner to seal in her rose lipstick, preventing bleeding. A soft, matte brown eye shadow on the upper lid created depth and made her blue eyes pop. Or should I say *detonate*!

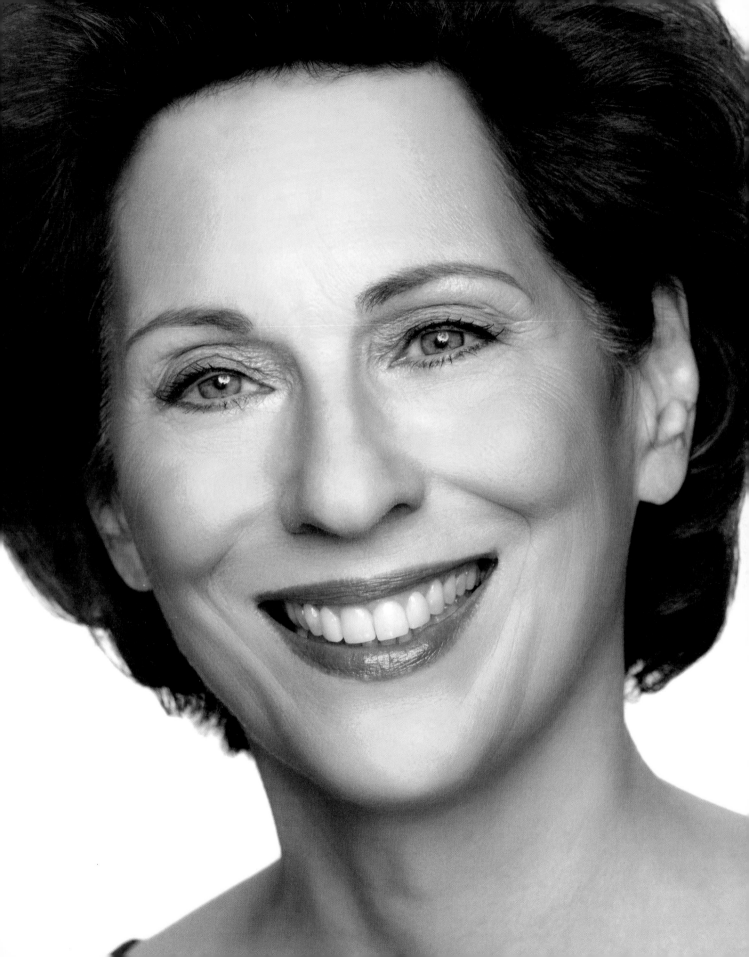

Bernice, 18

My parents feel I should focus on my studies, not my looks. If you saw pictures of my junior high makeup experiments, you'd agree with them.

I used to wear the weirdest eye shadows and heavy foundation. Once I ripped out all my lashes after tangling with a curler. I think I've now found the right balance—no more raccoon eyes!

When I was little, people used to pinch my nose—pointing out how there's no bridge, unlike Western noses. But now I accept myself and am happy with how I look. My boyfriend thinks my nose is cute and says my smile is contagious!

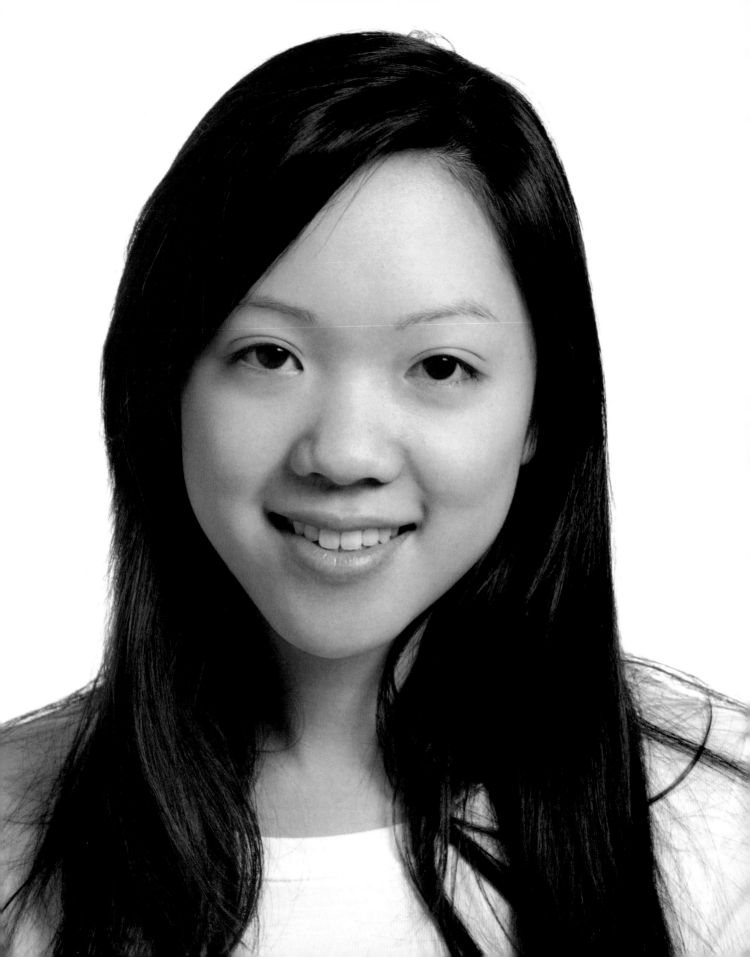

Carmindy Vision: What I See

When I see Asian women, I immediately think of them as naturally blessed with so many beautiful assets: smooth skin, full lips, exotic eyes. I never realized the nose bridge issue until Bernice mentioned it. Let's drop corrosive comparisons like East versus West and get busy celebrating unique beauty!

Bernice has such doll-like porcelain skin, I decided to go for a youthful, romantic look.

On her eyes, I used a shimmering white highlight under the brow, a granite shadow to define the lash line, and a taupe shadow across the lid. Using a corner lash curler, we lifted her lashes and applied a healthy dose of black mascara. We also defined her brows to frame her entire face.

To accentuate her creamy complexion, I applied a pretty pink blush. A slick of pale pink lip gloss played up her beautiful coloring. Exquisite!

Paula, 35

HOMETOWN: SAN JUAN, PUERTO RICO

I first decided to change my look in seventh grade, when I asked for a really short haircut. It wasn't a wise choice. For a long time after that, I felt I couldn't trust my beauty instincts. I went in search of women to emulate instead of seeing and bringing out my unique assets.

As I got older and grew professionally, I came into my own physically as well. Now I make an effort to look pulled together as Paula, not as a carbon copy of my friends or cousins. I know how much better I feel when I don't just rush out the door, but take a moment to apply makeup and be at my best. I have my routine down to ten minutes flat!

Today I feel most beautiful when I'm enjoying myself—just by being around the right people, whether they're coworkers, friends, or family. When I can just be myself, I drop any self-consciousness and love living in the moment.

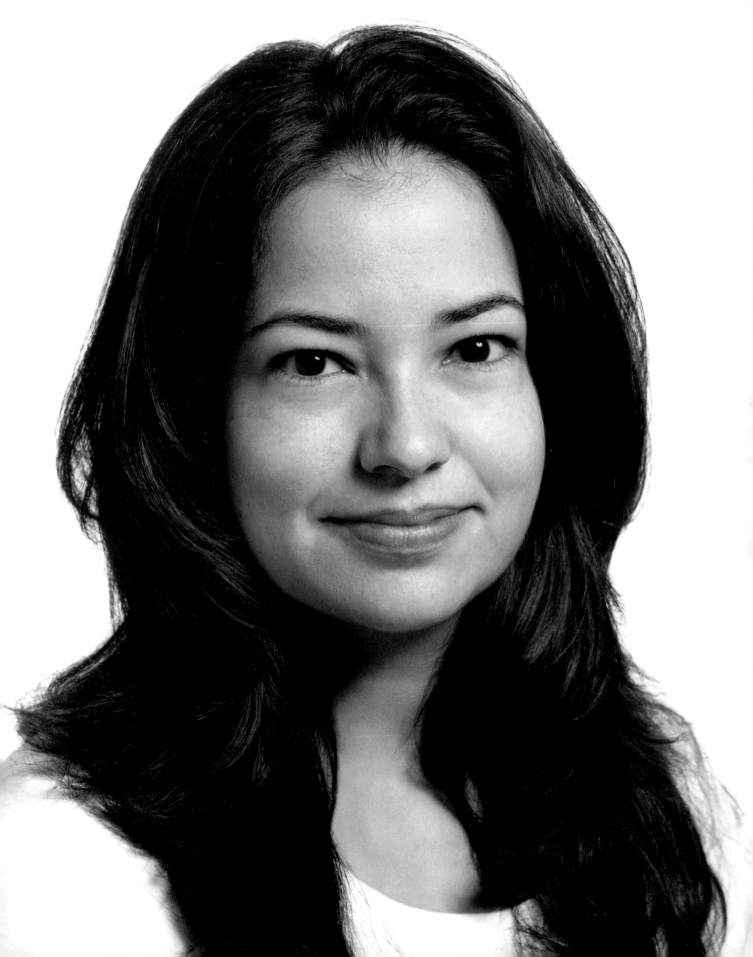

Carmindy Vision: What I See

Paula's face lights up the room. Her smile is contagious, topped only by her laugh. Everything about her says here's a vivacious, happy, deeply confident woman.

To highlight her sunny personality, I went for a summery, fresh look.

We defined her eyes using a bronze shimmer in the crease, with sunset gold and pink shadows under the brow and across the lid. A sweep of bronze shadow under the lower lash line brought out the sparkle. We curled her lashes and added black mascara to fire up the flirt factor.

Brights enhanced Paula's honey complexion. We played up her Latina coloring with coral powder blush and coral lip gloss. Absolutely radiant!

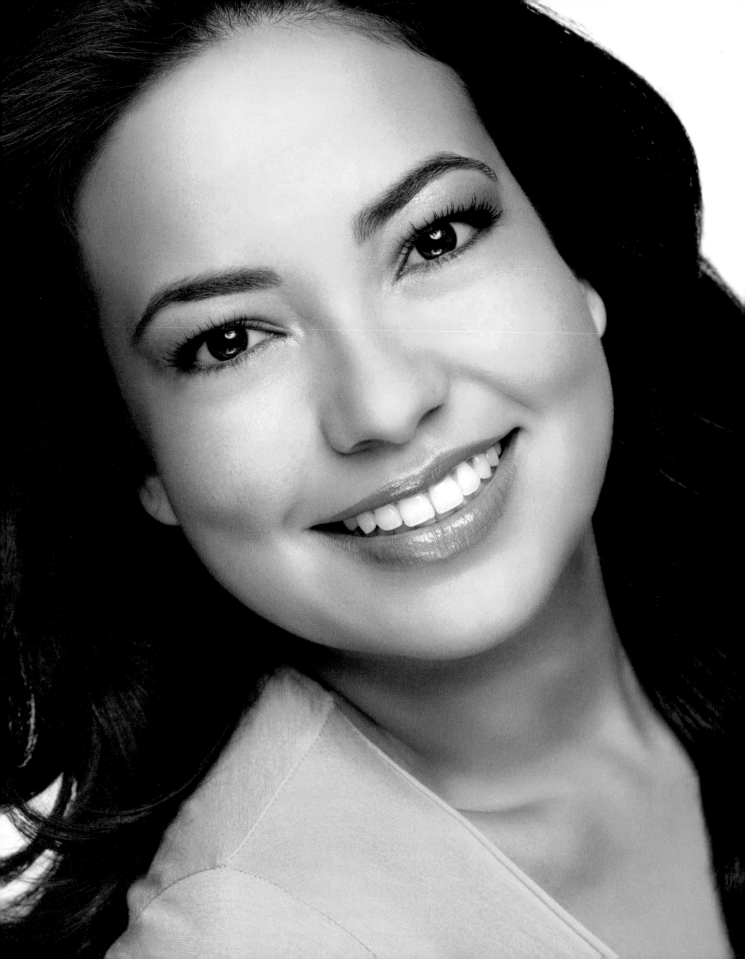

Heather, 22

HOMETOWN: BENSALEM, PENNSYLVANIA

I can't remember ever not being aware of the importance of appearance. I've always been taller and curvier than most girls. And for that stretch from twelve to sixteen, I felt quite a mess: I had braces, felt "big" among my peers, and boys would refer to my round cheeks as "fat face."

When those braces came off, however, I felt a glow of happy white light. People tell me I have a great smile, so the investment paid off.

Every year I feel better about my looks. Sometimes negative self-talk still creeps in. I think my nose, ears, and lips are asymmetrical. Crooked, in fact! Hopefully those hang-ups will pass in time, too.

I once read that a girl becomes a woman when she can accept a compliment. As I move into adulthood, I try to remember that.

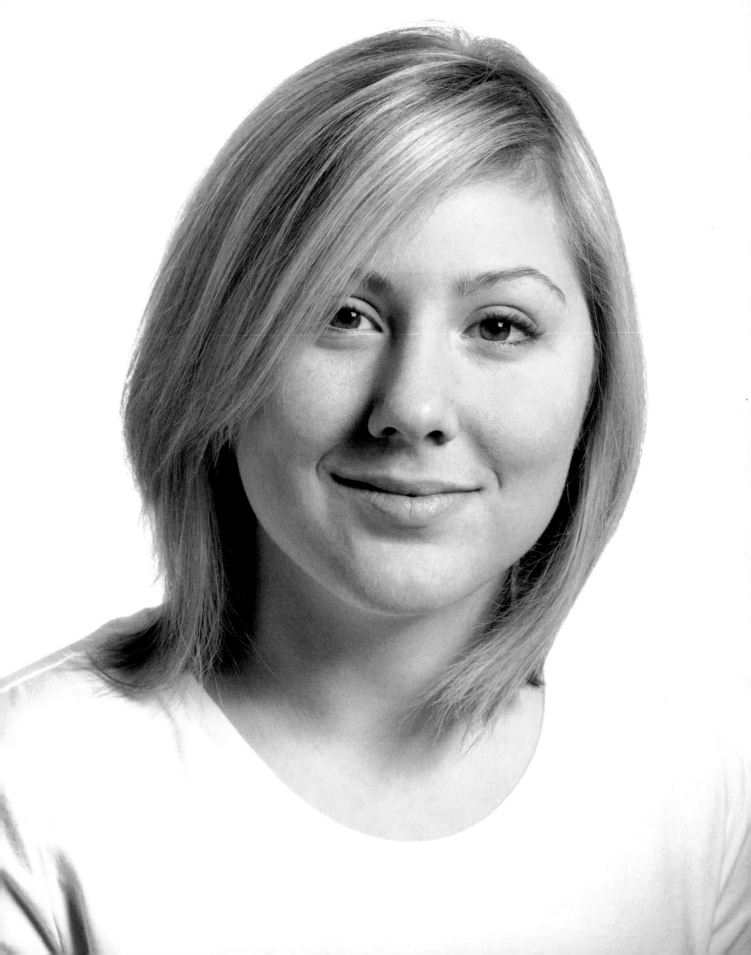

Carmindy Vision: What I See

Of all my makeover ladies, Heather and I have the most in common. Those taunts about our round faces have stuck with us for too long. What a waste of energy. I mean, come on!

Heather has a classically beautiful face with porcelain skin, a radiant smile, and a natural rosy blush on those cheeks. She just screams youthful vitality! I can't wait to see her grow more comfortable in her own beauty.

To highlight her sunny personality, I went with a golden look for Heather. We swept bronzer on her cheeks, forehead, and temples. To play up her soft brown eyes, I chose gold and copper shadows and finished with a sweep of black mascara. A nude, high-shine gloss was all her high-wattage smile required. Luminous!

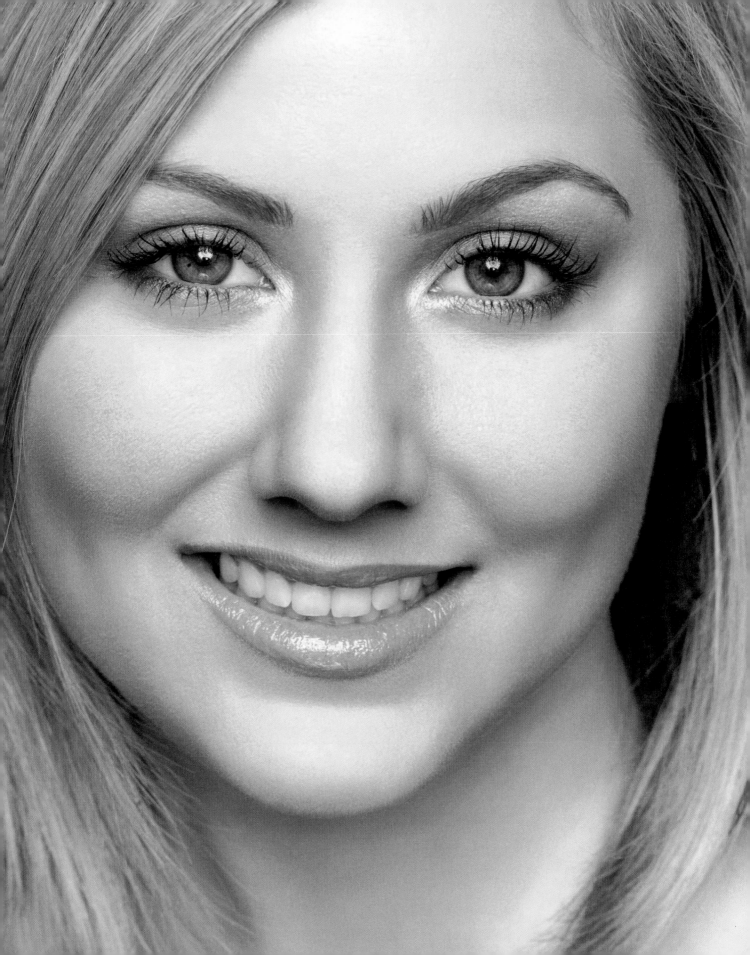

Elise, 47, and Alexa, 13

HOMETOWN: NEW YORK, NEW YORK

Alexa: At thirteen, I don't want to look like a baby, but I'm not sure about makeup technique. I do know I want to look genuine and down-to-earth. Too many girls just pack it on. I'm not into that.

Elise: I hope to set a good example for Alexa. I used to see myself as "just cute" (I'm five feet), but now, at forty-seven, I feel this is the best I've ever looked. As you mature, you learn how to best take care of yourself.

Nowadays I feel most beautiful when I'm being physically active, really expending energy, and then have the pleasure of relaxing in that post-exercise glow. You have to be inside your own beauty; that's when it really radiates.

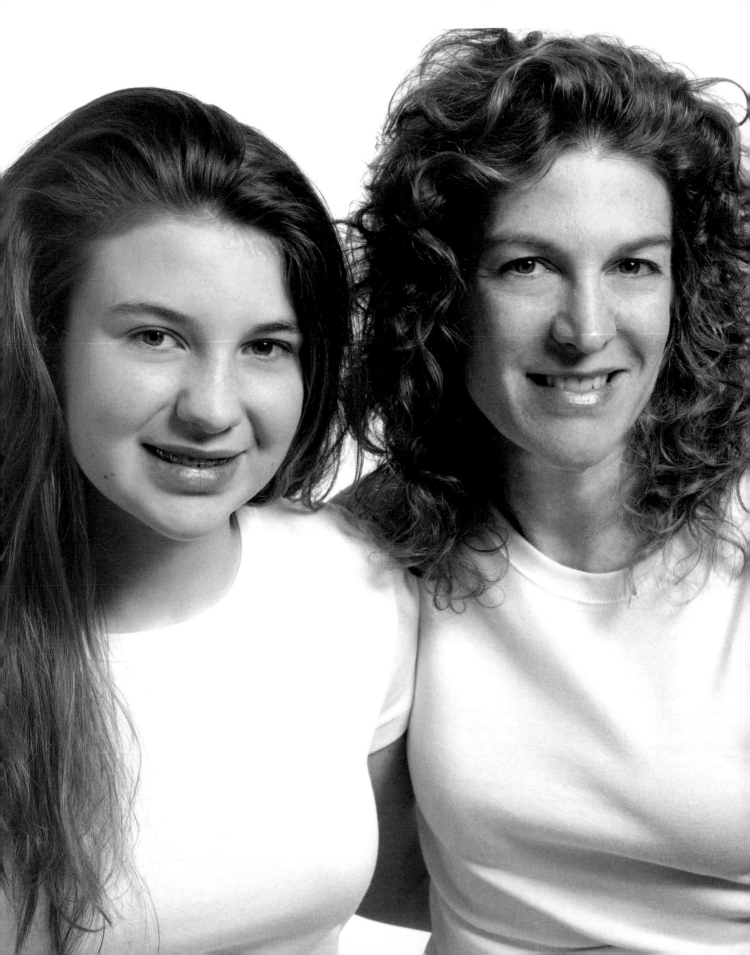

Carmindy Visioin: What I See

Alexa's eyes are true almond loveliness, and her skin is just terrific. As a young lady just starting to experiment, she should definitely leave her brows alone and be very light-handed with makeup.

I placed just a little iridescent shimmer shadow on her eyes, plus a sweep of black mascara. Pinky blush and lip color set off Alexa's sweet teen beauty.

Elise has cheekbones to die for—truly supermodel bone structure on her entire face. But she was confused about the right color palette to play up her features.

We started with a sheer application of liquid foundation to even out her skin and restored its vibrancy with some coral cream blush on the apples of her cheeks. For Elise's hazel eyes, we used khaki shadow and forest green liquid liner to bring out the irises' gold flecks. A neutral moisturizing lip color let her mouth's pretty shape stand on its own.

It was so wonderful to see a mother and daughter bloom with love and admiration right before our eyes. Inspiring!

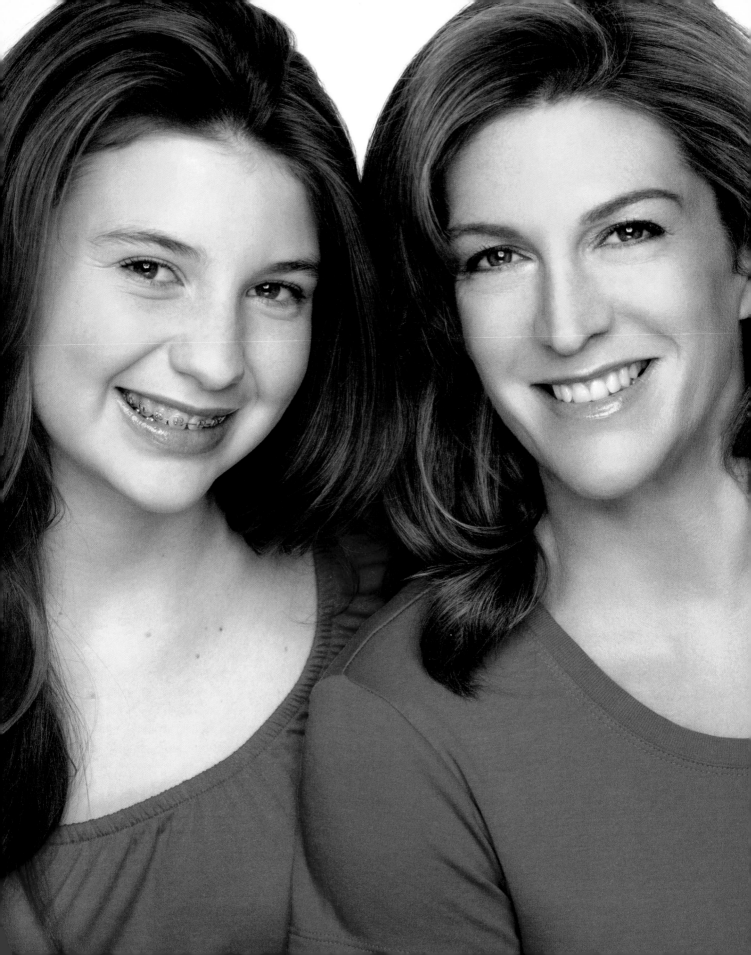

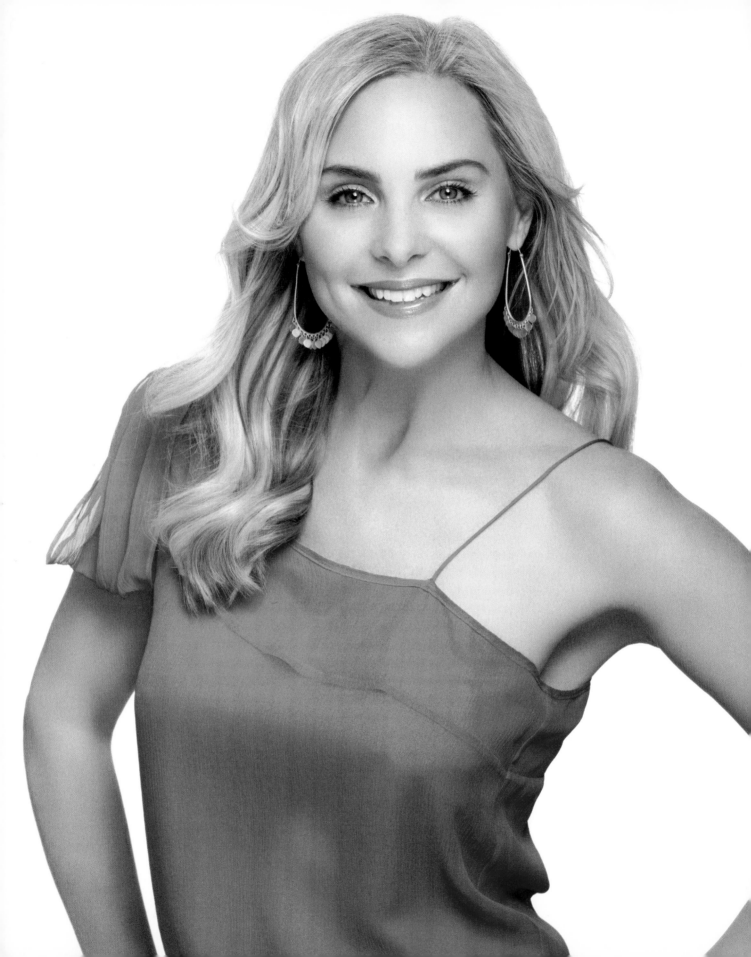

chapter fourteen *you are positively*
beautiful

Well, darlin', my publishers tell me our time together must come to an end. I hope you've enjoyed using this book as much as I've loved putting it together.

Rather than an ending, let's see this as a new beginning. After all, your beauty journey is just getting started! You're gaining positive momentum. And you're looking better every day because you're feeling better about your unique beauty—inside and out.

Congratulations! Take a moment to appreciate how far you've come.

You've dropped the flaw focus, embraced your assets, and enhanced your best features.

You're determined to end negative self-talk, and you're eager to spread the contagious joy of compliments.

You see yourself as one of a kind, glorious, and downright gorgeous.

And you know what? You're *right*.

LOVE, *Carmindy*

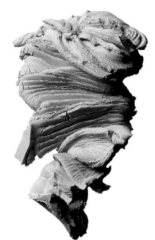
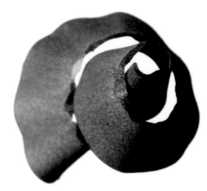
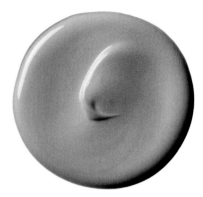
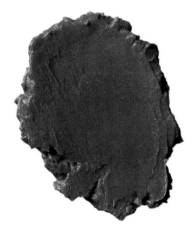
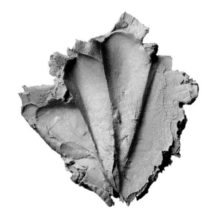
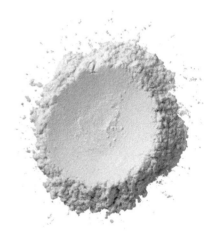
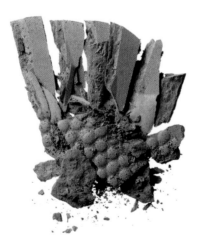
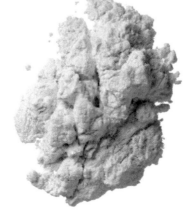
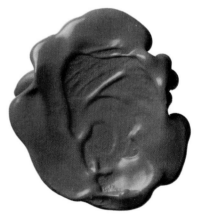

*shopping*guide

The following products are the best of the best. Over the years I have tried every product and every brand out there and I know what works. Here is your chance to peek inside my makeup bag. No matter what your budget is, you will find everything you need to get positively beautiful.

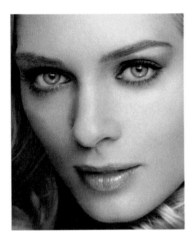

The Eyes Have It

Liquid Eyeliner

$$$ T LeClerc Liquid Eyeliner

$ Sally Hansen Natural Beauty Inspired by Carmindy Always Perfect Liquid Eyeliner

Waterproof Liquid Eyeliner

$$$ MAC Liquidlast Liner

$ Maybelline Lineworks Liquid Eyeliner

Pencil Eyeliner

$$$ Chanel Le Crayon Khol Intense Eye Pencil

$ Styli-Style Line & Blend Square Eye Pencil

Waterproof Pencil Eyeliner

$$$ Urban Decay 24/7 Glide-On Eye Pencil

$ NYC Waterproof Eyeliner Pencil

Highlight Pencil Eyeliner

$$$ Paula Dorf Eye Liner in Enhancer

$ Rimmel London Soft Kohl Kajal Eye Pencil in Pure White

Powder Eye Shadow

$$$ Dior Eyeshadow Sets

$ Sally Hansen Natural Beauty Inspired by Carmindy Instant Definition Eye Shadow Palette

Cream Eye Shadow

$$$ Benefit Creaseless Cream Shadow/Liner

$ Rimmel London All Day Wear Cream Eyeshadow

Mascara

$$$ Kanebo Styling Mascara

$ Sally Hansen Natural Beauty Inspired by Carmindy Lift and Define Mascara

Tube Technology Mascara

$$$ Blinc Kiss Me Mascara

$ Not available at press time

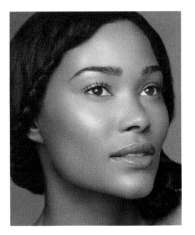

Skin Deep

Primer

$$$ Smashbox Photo Finish Foundation Primer

$ Sally Hansen Natural Beauty Inspired by Carmindy
Luminizing Face Primer

Liquid Foundation

$$$ Make Up For Ever Face & Body Liquid Makeup

$ Sally Hansen Natural Beauty Inspired by Carmindy Your Skin Makeup

Tinted Moisturizer

$$$ LORAC ProtecTINT SPF 30 Oil-Free Tinted Moisturizer

$ Neutrogena Healthy Skin Glow Sheers

Spray Foundation

$$$ Classified Cosmetics ERA FACE Spray-on Foundation

$ Sally Hansen Airbrush Makeup SPF 8

Cream Foundation

$$$ La Mer The Treatment Crème Foundation SPF 15

$ CoverGirl Advanced Radiance Restorative Cream Foundation

Under-Eye Concealer

$$$ Amazing Cosmetics Amazing Concealer

$ Sally Hansen Natural Beauty Inspired by Carmindy
Fast Fix Concealer

Pressed Powder

$$$ MAC Blot Powder

$ Sally Hansen Natural Beauty Inspired by Carmindy
Luminous Matte Pressed Powder

Loose Powder

$$$ T LeClerc Loose Powder

$ Sally Hansen Natural Beauty Inspired by Carmindy Truly
Translucent Loose Powder

Cream Highlighter

$$$ Fresh Satin Luster Face Palette

$ Wet n Wild MegaGlo Face Illuminator

Powder Highlighter

$$$ MAC Pigment Powder (in lightest shades)

$ NYC Sparkle Eye Dust (great for cheekbones, too)

Cream Bronzer

$$$ NARS The Multiple

$ Sally Hansen Natural Beauty Inspired by Carmindy
Sheerest Cream Bronzer

Powder Bronzer

$$$ Guerlain Terracotta Bronzing Powder

$ Sally Hansen Natural Beauty Inspired by Carmindy Sun
Glow Powder Bronzer

Spray Bronzer

$$$ Classified Cosmetics ERA RAYZ Spray On Bronzer

$ Sally Hansen Airbrush Shimmer

Cleanser

$$$ La Mer The Cleansing Gel

$ Cetaphil Gentle Skin Cleanser

Drying Lotion

$$$ Bliss Change Your Spots

$ Clearasil Ultra Acne Treatment Cream, Vanishing

See the "Beauty for Every Season" section for other product recommendations mentioned in chapter six, "Skin Deep."

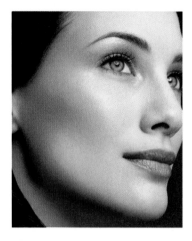

Getting Cheeky

Powder Blush

$$$ Lancôme Blush Subtil

$ Sally Hansen Natural Beauty Inspired by Carmindy
Natural Powder Blush

Cream Blush

$$$ Benefit Sheer Cream Blusher

$ Sally Hansen Natural Beauty Inspired by Carmindy
Sheerest Cream Blush

Gel Blush

$$$ Clinique Gel Blush

$ Revlon Pinch Me Sheer Gel Blush

Stain Blush

$$$ Benefit Benetint

$ The Body Shop Lip & Cheek Stain

For highlighter and bronzer see the list under "Skin Deep."

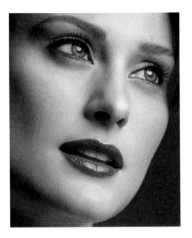

Luscious Lips

Colored Lip Liner

$$$ Guerlain Lip Pencil

$ NYC Automatic Lipliner

Highlight Lip Liner

$$$ Guerlain Divinora Lip Pencil in Cupidon

$ CoverGirl CG Eyeslicks in Cream Soda (highlights lips, too)

Lipstick

$$$ Lipstick Queen Lipstick

$ Sally Hansen Natural Beauty Inspired by Carmindy Color
Comfort Lip Color

Lip Gloss

$$$ Giorgio Armani Lip Gloss

$ Sally Hansen Natural Beauty Inspired by Carmindy Natural
Shine Lip Gloss

Tinted Lip Balm

$$$ Bobbi Brown Tinted Lip Balm

$ Sally Hansen Natural Beauty Inspired by Carmindy Moisture Plump Lip Balm

Stains

$$$ Benefit Benetint (also great on cheeks)

$ Revlon Just Bitten Lip Stain

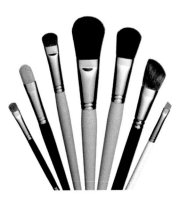

Tool Time

Slanted-Edge Tweezers

$$$ Tweezerman Slant Tweezer

$ La Cross Exacta Tweeze-Tapered Slant

Pointed-Edge Tweezers

$$$ Tweezerman Point Tweezer

$ La Cross Exacta Tweeze-Needlepoint

Scissors

$$$ Anastasia Brow Scissors

$ La Cross Cuticle Scissors-Ultra-Fine Point

Brow Brush

$$$ Paula Dorf Brow Groomer Brush

$ Posh Comb/Eyebrow Groomer

Angled Brow Brush

$$$ Benefit Hard Angle Brush

$ Posh Brushes Brow Brush

Nonlatex Sponges

$$$ Cover FX Non Latex Wedge Sponges

$ Posh Brushes 32ct Non Latex Wedges

Under-Eye Concealer Brush

$$$ Vincent Longo #25 Concealer Brush

$ Essence of Beauty Synthetic Conceal Brush

Small-Tipped Concealer Brush

$$$ Shu Uemura Synthetic Brush 5F

$ Posh Brushes Fine Conceal & Touch Up Brush

Blush Brush

$$$ Body & Soul Brush #1

$ Essence of Beauty Pure Powder Brush Face

Powder Brush

$$$ Body & Soul Brush #2

$ Posh Brushes Blush Brush (use for powder)

Fan Brush

$$$ Benefit Fantail Brush

$ Jane Iredale White Fan Brush

Bronzer Brush

$$$ MAC #169 Angled Brush

$ Essence of Beauty Angle Powder Brush

Double-Ended Highlighter Brush

$$$ Stila #30 Double Ended Shadow Brush

$ Essence of Beauty Dual Use Eye Shadow Brush

Angled Eyeliner Brush

$$$ MAC #266 Small Angle Brush

$ Balm shadyLady Liner Brush

Liquid Transformer

$$$ Paula Dorf Transformer

$ La Femme Cake Eyeliner Sealer

Lid Eye Shadow Brush

$$$ Body & Soul Brush #4

$ Essence of Beauty Dual Use Eye Shadow Brush

Crease Eye Shadow Brush

$$$ Body & Soul Brush #3

$ Essence of Beauty Crease Brush Duo Eyes

Corner Lash Curler

$$$ Japonesque Precision Lash Curler, Metal

$ Tweezerman Corner Lash Curler

Metal Lash Comb

$$$ Profaces Metal Lash Comb

$ Tweezerman Folding llashcomb

Lip Brush

$$$ Shu Uemura Synthetic Brush 6F

$ Posh Brushes Retractable Lip Brush

Sharpener

$$$ Make Up For Ever Double Barrel Pencil Sharpener

$ Posh Brushes Duo Sharpener

Blotting Papers

$$$ Bourjois Anti-Shine Blotting Sheets

$ Clean & Clear Oil Absorbing Sheets

Brush Cleaner

$$$ Cinema Secrets Professional Brush Cleaner

$ Brush Off Makeup Brush Cleanser

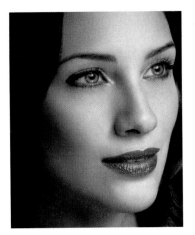

Beauty for Every Season

Sunscreen

$$$ Skin Ceuticals Physical UV Defense SPF 30

$ Neutrogena Ultra Sheer Dry-Touch Sunblock SPF 55

Self-Tanner

$$$ Clarins Self Tanning Instant Gel

$ Neutrogena MicroMist Tanning Sunless Spray

Mattifying Gel

$$$ OC Eight Professional Mattifying Gel

$ Good Skin All Right Mattifying Gel

Winter Skin Cream

$$$ Crème de la Mer

$ Avon ANEW RETROACTIVE + Youth Extending Cream Night

Eye Cream

$$$ La Mer The Eye Balm

$ Garnier Nutritioniste Ultra-Lift Anti-Wrinkle Firming Eye Cream

Healing Lip Balm

$$$ by Terry Rose Balm

$ Rosebud Perfume Co. Smith's Rosebud Salve

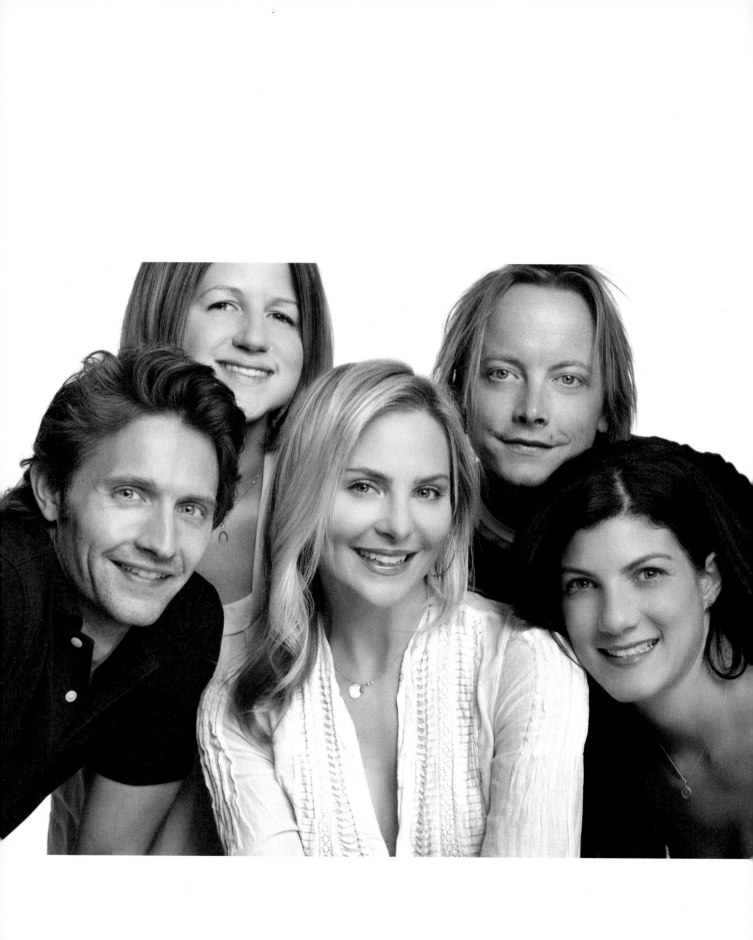

acknowledgments

These fabulous people shared this beautiful book experience with me, and I am truly blessed to have them in my life. Thank you all for your hard work and belief in the power of positive change.

Lauren Keller Galit—Powerhouse agent, support system, and friend who never ceases to amaze me. Thank you from the bottom of my heart.

Jay Sternberg and Gay Feldman—My agents/managers/extended family. You have showered me with love and light, protected me, and helped me grow. I love you.

Joy Bergmann—Where do I begin? You are a supervixen of words, a truly magical and beautiful woman. This book is as much of you as it is of me. We are the dream team. Kitchen Table Productions forever!

Sarah Sper and Center Street Books—Thank you for your joyful excitement and for giving me the opportunity to help women realize their beauty.

Peter Buckingham—The dreamiest photographer ever. Your incredible talent and energy radiates from these pages. You made these women feel like goddesses.

Edgar Mata, Brandon Harman, and Jean Bourbon—Peter's posse, who helped create the magic.

Noah Hatton—My friend and a hairstylist from heaven. Your love of women, passion for hair, and attention to detail created a frame of natural beauty.

Devon Jarvis—A creative genius and still-life extraordinaire. You simply are the best!

Daya Marron—Wardrobe stylist and dear friend. You did such an amazing job and made everyone feel comfortable and confident.

Lulu Chen—My fabulous stylist. Thank you for always getting it and making me look so darn good.

Emily Kate Warren—My lovely makeup assistant, who kept me organized and laughing. You are wonderful.

Erica Cruz—Thank you for your undying devotion and dedication. As my personal assistant, your patience and integrity is forever appreciated. Your beauty and light is a gift.

My gorgeous models and friends: Katherine Atkinson, Joy Bergmann, Sarah Burningham, Ivonne Casas, Dana Douglas, Marie Claude Jones, Lucy Kemp, Alexa and Elise Leopold, Cassie Lewis, Khrystine Muldowney, Michelle Oliver, Paula Rosado, Lois Safian, Heather Saltzman, and Bernice Wong. You are positively beautiful!!!

My fans—You lent your wisdom and asked the questions real women wanted answered, ensuring this book would be relevant and inspiring. We loved reading every one of your hundreds of e-mails!

Darbin Navarro and Danielle Borgia at Sun Studios—You greeted us every morning with a warm smile and hot tea. Thank you for your continued encouragement.

Thanks also to the wonderful people at Miguelina (www.miguelina.com) and Barneys New York for all the beautiful clothes.

My fantastic jewelry is courtesy of Me&Ro (www.meandrojewelry.com), Meira T (www.meiratdesigns.com), and Lena Skadegard, available at Christopher Totman (212-925-7495).

Finally, a very special, sugar-coated thank you to my wonderful family: Jack, Julie, and Quinn Bowyer. I love you.

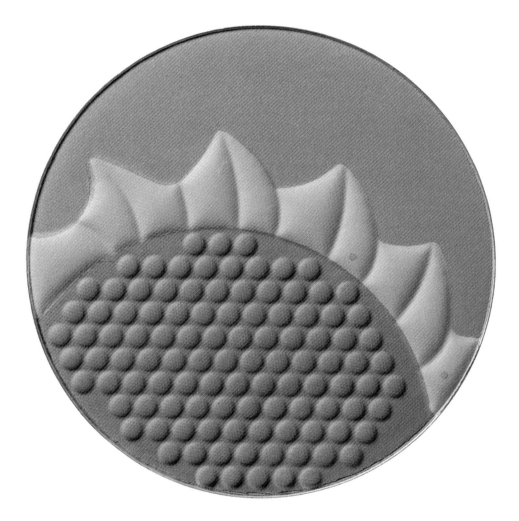

CARMINDY was raised in Southern California, where she started doing makeup fifteen years ago. Today she is the makeup artist on TLC's #1 show *What Not to Wear* and has appeared on the *Today Show*, *CBS Sunday Morning*, CBN, as well as in the *New York Times*, *Cosmopolitan*, *Elle*, *O*, *Glamour*, *Self*, *Lucky*, *GQ*, *Essence*, *Details*, *Marie Claire*, and *InStyle*. She lives in New York City with her husband.

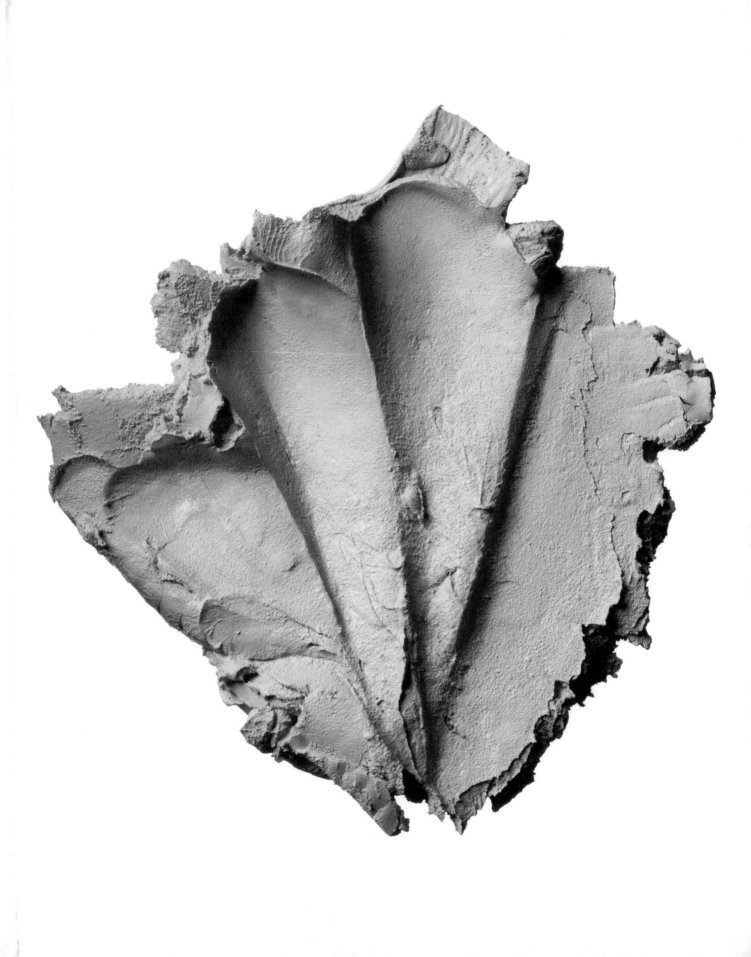

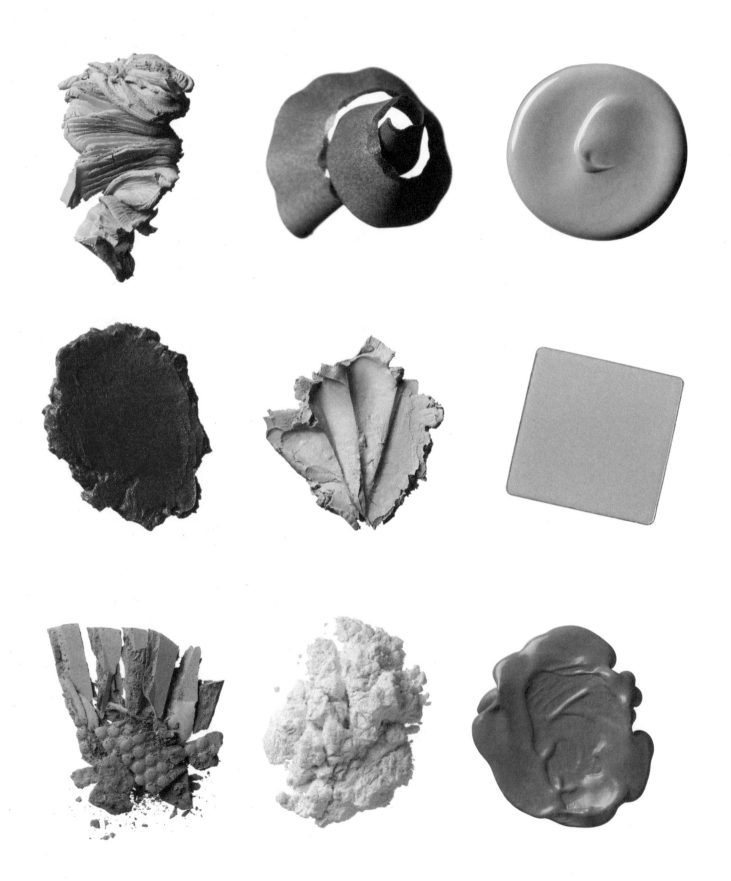